Mayo Clinic on Hearing

Wayne Olsen, Ph.D.

Editor in Chief

Mayo Clinic
Rochester, Minnesota

Mayo Clinic on Hearing provides reliable information about preserving your hearing and coping with hearing loss. Much of the information comes directly from the experience of health care professionals at Mayo Clinic. This book supplements the advice of your personal physician, whom you should consult for individual medical problems. *Mayo Clinic on Hearing* does not endorse any company or product. MAYO, MAYO CLINIC, MAYO CLINIC HEALTH INFORMATION and the Mayo triple-shield logo are marks of Mayo Foundation for Medical Education and Research.

Hardcover Library Edition Published 2004
Mason Crest Publishers
370 Reed Road
Suite 302
Broomall, PA 19008-0914
(866) MCP-BOOK (toll free)

First Printing

1 2 3 4 5 6 7 8 9 10

Library of Congress Catalog Card Number: 2003107354

ISBN 1-59084-805-5

Photo credits: Cover photos and the photos on pages 1, 11, 22, 23, 67 and 83 are from PhotoDisc®; photo on page 60 courtesy of Bacou-Dalloz Hearing Protection; photos on page 98 courtesy of Paws With A Cause.

Printed in the United States of America

About hearing loss

Many of us live in a noisy world that only seems to get noisier. We are assaulted daily by the roar and clatter of automobile traffic, jet airplanes, heavy equipment, home appliances and booming amplifiers and stereo systems. All this noise takes a toll on our ears.

Hearing loss is the third most common chronic condition in the United States. An estimated one-third of Americans older than age 65 and one-half of those older than age 75 are living with a hearing impairment. But you don't have to live in a world of muted, less distinct sounds. Steps that you and your physician or audiologist can take may improve what you hear.

The thirteenth book in Mayo's On Health series, *Mayo Clinic on Hearing*, provides you with clear explanations of the hearing exam, many common hearing problems and strategies to manage hearing loss in your daily life. The content is amply illustrated with drawings and photographs to enhance the text. A glossary and listing of additional resources are included at the back of the book.

About Mayo Clinic

Mayo Clinic evolved from the frontier practice of Dr. William Worrall Mayo and the partnership of his two sons, William J. and Charles H. Mayo, in the early 1900s. Pressed by the demands of their busy practice in Rochester, Minn., the Mayo brothers invited other physicians to join them, pioneering the private group practice of medicine. Today, with more than 2,000 physicians and scientists at its three major locations in Rochester, Minn., Jacksonville, Fla., and Scottsdale, Ariz., Mayo Clinic is dedicated to providing comprehensive diagnoses, accurate answers and effective treatments.

With this depth of medical knowledge, experience and expertise, Mayo Clinic occupies an unparalleled position as a health information resource. Since 1983 Mayo Clinic has published reliable health information for millions of consumers through award-winning newsletters, books and online services. Revenue from the publishing activities supports Mayo Clinic programs, including medical education and research.

Editorial staff

Editor in Chief
Wayne Olsen, Ph.D.

Managing Editor
Kevin Kaufman

Copy Editor
Mary Duerson

Proofreading
Miranda Attlesey
Donna Hanson

Editorial Research
Anthony Cook
Dana Gerberi
Deirdre Herman
Michelle Hewlett

Contributing Writers
Lee Engfer
Rachel Haring

Creative Director
Daniel Brevick

Art Director
Paul Krause

Illustration and Photography
Richard Madsen
Kent McDaniel
Christopher Srnka
Rebecca Varga

Medical Illustration
Michael King

Indexing
Larry Harrison

Contributing editors and reviewers

Ann Anderson, M.S.
Christopher Bauch, Ph.D.
Charles Beatty, M.D.
Robert Brey, Ph.D.
Michael Cevette, Ph.D.
Jodi Cook, Ph.D.
Melissa DeJong, M.A.
Colin Driscoll, M.D.

George Facer, M.D.
Christopher Frye
Stephen Harner, M.D.
David Hawkins, Ph.D.
Jennifer Jacobson
Larry Lundy, M.D.
Martin Robinette, Ph.D.
Jon Shallop, Ph.D.

Preface

Hearing loss is the third most common medical problem in the United States. For some, hearing loss is present at birth or is hereditary. More commonly, hearing loss is a complication of illness and disease, powerful or excess medication, exposure to loud sounds and the normal process of aging. Commonsense precautions, such as using hearing protection when exposed to loud sounds, often can help you avoid or at least reduce the problems associated with hearing loss.

This book describes the delicate, sensitive structures of the human ear. Attention is focused on many common ear disorders and the ear-related problems of tinnitus and dizziness. Explanations are provided for diagnostic tests, medical treatment, surgery, and other forms of remediation. This information can help you appreciate the exquisite function of your ears and understand the cause of a hearing problem. It also allows for a more informed participation by you in prevention or treatment strategies.

Medical treatment or surgery generally can resolve ear discomfort and sometimes improve hearing. But when hearing loss cannot be alleviated medically, an array of electronic and digital devices is available to help you hear better and communicate more easily. The selection and use of hearing aids, cochlear implants and assistive listening devices are discussed in separate chapters.

Audiologists and ear, nose and throat specialists at Mayo Clinic facilities in Rochester, Minn., Jacksonville, Fla., and Scottsdale, Ariz., have reviewed the content of this book for accuracy and completeness. The result is a concise, practical resource to assist you in preserving your hearing, in functioning well in difficult listening situations and in minimizing the impact of hearing problems on your daily life.

Wayne Olsen, Ph.D.
Editor in Chief

Contents

Preface   v

Part 1: Understanding common hearing problems

Chapter 1	**How you hear**	3
	Structure of the ear	4
	Characteristics of sound	8
	Sound pathways	10
	Types of hearing loss	13
	Compensating for hearing loss	15
Chapter 2	**Getting a hearing exam**	17
	Who provides ear care?	18
	Who should have a hearing exam?	20
	What's involved in a hearing exam?	21
	Understanding your audiogram	32
	Taking action	34
Chapter 3	**Common problems of the outer ear and middle ear**	35
	Outer ear problems	36
	Eardrum problems	40
	Middle ear problems	43
Chapter 4	**Common problems of the inner ear**	53
	Presbycusis	54
	Noise-induced hearing loss	56
	Sudden deafness	59
	Other causes of hearing loss	60
	Research on the horizon	69

Chapter 5 **Tinnitus**   71

Unraveling a mystery   72

Types   73

Diagnosis   76

Management   77

Part 2: The management of hearing loss

Chapter 6 **Living with hearing impairment**   85

Hearing loss and quality of life   86

Strategies for social interaction   92

Finding support   99

Chapter 7 **Hearing aids**   103

Setting priorities and realistic expectations   104

How a hearing aid works   106

Selecting a hearing aid   107

Purchasing a hearing aid   114

Adjusting to a hearing aid   118

Taking care of your hearing aid   123

Chapter 8 **Cochlear implants**   125

Cochlear implants and hearing aids   126

How does a cochlear implant work?   127

Who can benefit from a cochlear implant?   128

Keeping your expectations realistic   129

Getting a cochlear implant   131

Adjusting to a cochlear implant   136

Staying positive   138

Chapter 9 **Other communication aids** 139

Difficult listening environments 140

Assistive listening devices 141

Telecommunications devices and services 147

Captioning 149

Alerting devices 150

On the horizon 151

Many options 153

Chapter 10 **Dizziness and problems with balance** 155

How does your balance system work? 156

Causes of dizziness 159

Diagnostic tests 160

Vestibular disorders 165

Vestibular rehabilitation 173

Additional resources 177

Glossary 181

Index 187

Part 1

Understanding common hearing problems

Chapter 1

How you hear

In 1802 Ludwig van Beethoven wrote a letter to his brothers expressing his innermost fears about deteriorating hearing: "Almost alone, and only mixing in society when absolutely necessary, I am compelled to live as an exile. If I approach near to people, a feeling of hot anxiety comes over me lest my condition should be noticed."[1] It's striking that such feelings belonged to a composer whose music, more than two centuries later, still brings so much listening enjoyment to people around the world.

But if you're experiencing problems with hearing, you, like Beethoven, may feel uncomfortable when you're in public. Not being able to hear clearly can be frustrating, to say the least, as you attempt to understand what others are telling you. It can cause social isolation when you find it easier to withdraw from conversations than to participate in them. Such behavior might in turn cause people to think of you as timid, arrogant or disconnected and to give up trying to communicate with you.

Then again, if you have hearing loss, you have plenty of company. At least 10 percent of Americans — 28 million — have some degree of hearing loss, ranging from mild to profound. Older adults are most affected, as hearing tends to deteriorate with age.

---

[1]Eaglefield-Hull, A., ed. *Beethoven's Letters*. New York: Dover; 1972: 38.

An estimated 30 percent of Americans age 65 and older, and approximately 50 percent of those over age 75, have a hearing impairment. But hearing loss can occur at any age due to factors such as noise exposure, trauma, genetics and illness. Worldwide, the number of people with hearing loss is estimated at 500 million.

Many people refuse to acknowledge their hearing loss. Only about one person in four who would benefit from a hearing aid actually wears one. Many choose to persevere without assistance. Yet people with hearing impairment who don't use hearing aids are more likely to feel sad or anxious, be less socially active and feel greater emotional insecurity than are those with hearing difficulties who do use hearing aids, according to a 1999 study from the National Council on Aging. The study also reported that hearing aid users have better relationships with their families.

Hearing aids have come a long way since the conspicuous ear trumpets of the 18th and 19th centuries. In fact, astounding improvements in hearing technology have been made in the last few decades. More options for treating hearing loss are available. And many of these options are less obvious to onlookers. The key is to find the treatment that's right for you.

In the chapters that follow, you'll find pertinent information about hearing loss — how it occurs, how it's diagnosed, how it can be treated and how you can live with it. You'll also learn about dizziness and problems with balance, conditions that sometimes are associated with hearing difficulties. With this knowledge you'll be better equipped to live an active, fulfilled life despite any changes that may occur to your hearing.

Structure of the ear

The ears are pretty amazing acoustic devices, as yet unmatched by human ingenuity. In a person with normal hearing, the ears, in combination with the brain, can almost instantly transform sound waves from the external world into the recognized voice of a loved one, the call of a songbird, a crack of thunder or the faint hum of an approaching vehicle.

Many factors play into this sensory wonder, so let's take a look at some of the important structures that make up the ear. The flap of cartilage on each side of your head may be the most recognizable structure, but that's only the external part of the ear. There are actually three complex, interconnected parts: the outer ear, middle ear and inner ear.

Outer ear

The outer ear is the part you can see sticking out from either side of your head. It's made up of folds of skin and cartilage, called the pinna (auricle), and the ear canal. The cup-like shape of the pinna (PIN-uh) gathers sound waves from the environment and directs them toward the ear canal.

The ear canal is an inch-long passageway leading to the eardrum (tympanic membrane). The skin lining the ear canal contains tiny hairs and glands that produce wax, or cerumen (suh-ROO-mun). The hairs and wax serve as a cleaning mechanism for the ear canal by repelling water, protecting against bacteria and keeping foreign objects such as dirt from slipping through the ear canal and reaching the eardrum. The eardrum is a thin, taut membrane that covers the entrance to the middle ear.

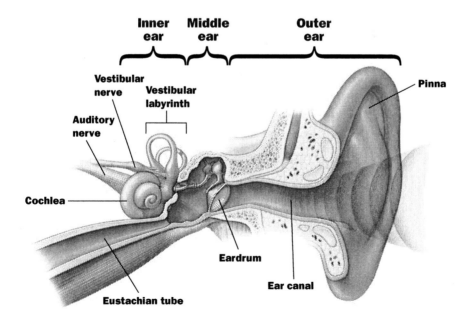

Middle ear

The middle ear is an air-filled cavity between the eardrum and the inner ear. The cavity is lodged in the temporal bone of your skull and houses three tiny bones called ossicles (OS-ih-kuls). The ossicles have scientific names, but each is commonly known by a name that describes its shape: the hammer (malleus), anvil (incus) and stirrup (stapes). Together, the ossicles form a bridge between the eardrum and the entrance of the inner ear (oval window). Each bone moves back and forth as a tiny lever to increase the sound level that reaches the inner ear. Two tiny muscles in the middle ear are attached to the hammer and the stirrup.

The middle ear provides access to the back of the nose and upper part of the throat, called the nasopharynx (nay-zo-FAIR-inks), through a narrow channel called the eustachian tube. The eustachian (u-STA-shun) tube normally remains closed until you swallow or yawn. Then it opens briefly to equalize the air pressure within your middle ear to the air pressure outside. You may feel and hear a pop when this occurs. Equal air pressure on both sides of the eardrum allows the membrane to vibrate easily.

In adults, the eustachian tube angles slightly down toward the nose and throat. In children, because their skull structures aren't yet fully developed, the eustachian tube is narrower and more horizontal. This makes it easier for a child's eustachian tube to become blocked and for fluid to build up behind the eardrum. Occasionally, this fluid becomes infected, causing a middle ear infection.

Structures of the middle ear

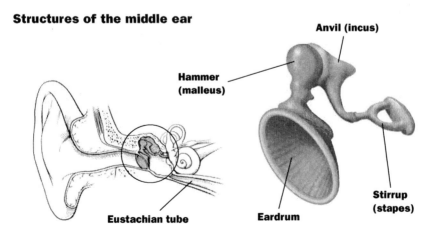

Anvil (incus)

Hammer (malleus)

Stirrup (stapes)

Eustachian tube

Eardrum

Inner ear

The inner ear contains the most sophisticated part of the hearing mechanism: the fluid-filled, snail-shaped cochlea (KOK-le-uh). The purpose of the cochlea is to translate incoming sound waves into electrical signals that can be understood by the brain.

The tube of the cochlea would be just over an inch in length if it were stretched out, but it naturally curls around almost three times. The whole structure is no bigger than about the size of a pea. The tube is divided into three chambers that spiral around a bony core: the upper chamber (scala vestibuli), the middle chamber or cochlear duct (scala media), and the lower chamber (scala tympani). The cochlear duct contains the organ of Corti, the organ responsible for hearing. Lining the organ of Corti is a strip of tissue called the basilar membrane, on which stand four rows of ultrasensitive hair cells topped by tiny tufts of fine hair strands (cilia and stereocilia). The tallest of these cilia are embedded in another membrane called the tectorial membrane.

The inner ear also contains a structure called the vestibular labyrinth, which assists your sense of balance. It consists of three semicircular tubes that, similar to the cochlea, are filled with fluid and contain hair cells sensitive to fluid movement. These cells track every movement of your body so that you're aware of where your head is in relation to the ground. Chapter 10 describes in greater detail the vestibular labyrinth and problems associated with it such as dizziness and vertigo.

Structures of the inner ear

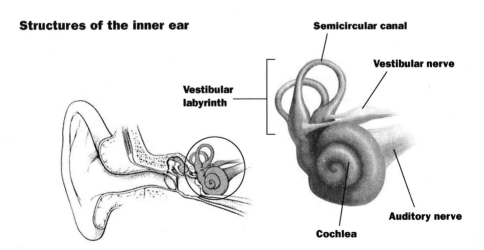

Semicircular canal

Vestibular nerve

Vestibular labyrinth

Auditory nerve

Cochlea

Characteristics of sound

The ear is a complex series of structures that enables you to collect and make sense of sound. But what is sound exactly? Sound occurs when something vibrates in matter. We hear objects that vibrate in the air, such as the oscillations of a person's voice box (larynx) that forms the patterns of speech or the pistons and belts of a running car engine. But sounds also travel through fluid such as water, for example, the acoustic echoes reflected off the ocean floor that are picked up by a sonar device on board a ship. Sounds also travel through solid matter such as bone or steel. The thump you hear when you bump your head against an object is a result of vibrations that travel through your skull, not the air.

When an object vibrates in matter, it displaces the molecules around it, in much the same way that a rock thrown into a pond causes the water to ripple in every direction. The vibration sends out a pressure wave. When a pressure wave travels through air to your outer ear and reaches your eardrum, it triggers a chain reaction in the middle ear, cochlea, auditory nerve and brain that allows you to hear the sound.

As you know, one sound can be vastly different from another. Think of the low-pitched rumble of a diesel truck and the high-pitched whine of a lightweight motorbike. Both sounds come from a type of combustion engine. But there's no mistaking one sound for the other. The differences between sounds arise mainly from three qualities — frequency, intensity and timbre. The first two qualities can be measured, and the third is subjective.

Frequency

The frequency of a sound, a quality also known as pitch, is how often a disturbed pressure wave fluctuates within a given period of time. This is usually measured in cycles per second, or hertz (Hz). The more fluctuations, the higher the frequency. Sound frequencies audible to humans range from around 20 Hz, a very low pitch, to 20,000 Hz, a very high pitch. Common sounds in human speech cover a broad range from about 250 Hz (a low-pitched vowel such as *ooo*) to around 4,000 Hz (a high-pitched consonant such as *sss*).

Intensity

The intensity of a sound is measured by its loudness (amplitude). This quality is associated with the level of disturbance in the pressure wave. It's measured in decibels (db). For example, a whisper might be measured at 30 decibels sound pressure level (db SPL), whereas a gunshot might register at 140 to 170 db SPL. Noises at the intensity level of a gunshot are too loud for the human ear to tolerate and can cause permanent damage if the ears aren't protected with earplugs or a hearing protective device (earmuffs). A subjective description of sound intensity is its loudness. For example, noises can be too soft, comfortably loud, too loud or painfully loud.

Sound pressure level and hearing level

Decibels are units of measure used to define the intensity of sound. Measuring the force of a sound wave in the environment or the amount of pressure it exerts on your eardrum is referred to as sound pressure level. The reference level of 0 decibels sound pressure level (db SPL) is about the weakest sound that can be heard with the best human ears. The intensity of normal speech is generally around 60 db SPL.

Decibels are units of measure that also establish how well your hearing compares with the average for a large group of young people with normal hearing. This measure is expressed in decibels hearing level (db HL). A person with a hearing threshold (the faintest point at which he or she can perceive sound) measured between 0 and 25 db HL is considered to have normal or near normal hearing. Someone who has trouble understanding conversational speech may barely hear sounds at 40 db HL but no lower. He or she would be considered to have moderate hearing loss. A person who can hear only a relatively loud voice close by may have a hearing threshold of 70 db HL and would have severe hearing loss.

In subsequent chapters a measure of intensity that is expressed in terms of *db* represents a measure of sound pressure level. When referring to a measure of hearing level, it will be expressed as *db HL*.

Timbre

Perhaps the most subjective aspect of sound is its timbre. Timbre is the quality that allows us to distinguish between sounds of the same frequency and intensity, such as the same note played by two different musical instruments or the enunciation of a vowel or consonant by two different voices.

Sound pathways

Sound is created by pressure waves moving through matter, and hearing is the perception of that sound. When you hear a sound, you perceive its qualities of frequency, intensity and timbre practically at once. The journey of a sound wave through the ear and to your brain may be instantaneous, but it is nonetheless complex.

It begins as the outer ear (pinna) gathers in sound waves and directs them toward your eardrum. Many mammals, such as cats and dogs, have the ability to rotate their outer ears to face the source of a sound. Humans don't have this ability. Instead, sound waves from different directions reach the pinna at different angles, at slightly different times and intensities, producing slightly different patterns depending on where the source of the sound is in relation to your head. This allows your brain to distinguish from where a voice is calling you.

Binaural hearing

Hearing with two ears is called binaural hearing. The use of both ears is critical to helping you locate the source of a sound. A sound occurring on your left will reach your left ear first and register as louder in your left ear than in your right. When your brain compares information from both ears, it can distinguish whether the sound originated from the left or the right.

In addition, your brain is able to distinguish sounds you want to hear and somewhat suppress background noise, with the help of auditory information arriving from both ears. An example of this function might be your ability to hold a conversation with someone at a crowded, noisy party.

Sound pathways

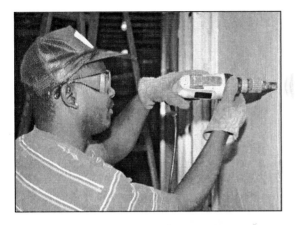

In the ear
Sound waves entering the ear travel through the ear canal and are transmitted as vibrations by the eardrum and ossicles to the inner ear. The vibrations cause a chemical reaction in the cochlea, triggering electrical impulses in the auditory nerve that are carried into the brain.

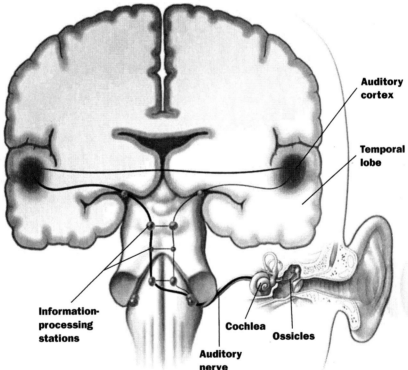

Auditory cortex

Temporal lobe

Information-processing stations

Cochlea

Ossicles

Auditory nerve

In the brain
The electrical impulses pass through and cross between several information-processing stations within the brain. Finally, the impulses end their path in the auditory cortex within the temporal lobes. There, the brain sorts, processes and files information about the sound.

Into the middle ear

After a sound wave travels through the ear canal, it strikes the taut membrane of the eardrum, causing the eardrum to vibrate. These vibrations cause the ossicles that bridge the space between the eardrum and the oval window — the entrance to the inner ear — to vibrate also. The ossicles move together like a tiny lever system. Because the surface of the eardrum is much larger than the oval window, the vibrations are delivered with greater force to the inner ear. Amplifying the sound increases the energy, which is necessary for the vibrations to travel through the fluid of the inner ear. Fluid offers more resistance than does air and thus requires a greater force to push through it.

If a sound is too loud, muscles in the middle ear constrict to reduce the effects of the sound and attempt to protect the inner ear. This is called an acoustic reflex. However, a sudden noise like a nearby gunshot can still cause immediate, permanent damage to the ear. That's because the auditory nerve must first respond to the sound before the muscles in the middle ear can contract, causing a slight delay.

Into the inner ear

The vibration of the stirrup against the oval window transmits the pattern of the sound wave to the inner ear and the fluid in the upper and lower galleries of the cochlea. The wave sets into motion the hair cells on the basilar membrane. Each frequency of the sound wave affects a specific section of the basilar membrane, thereby stimulating a response in the hair cells exactly at that location. If the sound has a very high frequency, the basilar membrane resonates with cells near the base of the cochlea. If the sound wave has a low frequency, the basilar membrane resonates closer to the tip of the cochlea.

The hair cells of the basilar membrane set in motion by the sound wave vibrate against the tectorial membrane. This motion displaces the cilia on the hair cells, resulting in a chemical reaction within the hair cells. This chemical reaction triggers electrical impulses in the auditory nerve. The louder or more intense the sound, the more impulses that are sent off.

Traveling to the brain

Electrical impulses travel through the auditory nerve to various information-processing centers within the brain. These circuits end in what's called the auditory cortex, located in the temporal lobes on each side of the brain. Commonly called gray matter because of its grayish, wrinkled appearance, the cortex is a thin layer of tissue where most of the brain's sorting, processing and filing of information is done. Passage of the impulses along twin circuits to the two auditory cortices is the grand finale of the hearing process.

The nerve impulses pass through a number of stations on their way to the auditory cortex. These stations begin processing the sounds to determine their origin. There's also plenty of communication between the right and left temporal lobes so that signals can be compared. The comparisons and analyses in the stations and auditory cortex also play a role in suppressing background noise and in allowing you to focus on the sounds you want to hear.

Scientists are still trying to understand how the brain interprets messages from the cochlea and identifies them as distinct sounds. At low frequencies the electrical impulses follow the same pattern of the sound waves. But at high frequencies the pattern varies.

Speech and language — how the brain gives meaning to sound — is associated closely with your ability to hear. We know that the process of storing and categorizing specific sounds in a person's memory starts at a young age. For example, at about 3 months, babies can differentiate their parents' voices from other voices. The study of speech and language is a growing field of research that may provide further insight into the mechanisms of hearing.

Types of hearing loss

One of the benefits scientists hope to gain by studying the mechanisms of hearing is the ability to help individuals whose hearing has been impaired. With such a complex auditory system, many small changes or slight damage to the ear can affect some or all of your hearing. Scientists have identified three types of hearing loss: conductive, sensorineural and mixed.

Conductive hearing loss

The ear canal and the middle ear conduct sound waves to the sensory receptors of your inner ear. If something blocks this pathway, sound can't get through properly, and the result is a reduced perception of sound. This can occur, for example, from excessive wax in the ear canal. Normally, your ear canal cleanses itself, but in some cases buildup occurs and may require professional removal. Other problems that can cause conductive hearing loss include foreign objects lodged in the ear, middle ear infections, head trauma and abnormal bone growth in the region of the ear. See Chapter 3 for more detailed information about conductive hearing loss.

Sensorineural hearing loss

Damage to the structures of the inner ear, such as the hair cells in the cochlea or the nerve fibers leading from the cochlea to the brain, can cause sensorineural (sen-suh-re-NOOR-ul) hearing loss. Such damage is most often associated with the general wear and tear of aging, known as presbycusis (pres-bih-KU-sis), or with excessive exposure to noise.

The initial damage is usually found at the base of the cochlea, where the basilar membrane responds to high frequencies. That's why people with sensorineural hearing loss often have trouble perceiving high-frequency sounds, such as certain consonants in speech. For example, someone with high-frequency hearing loss may be unable to distinguish *tell* from *sell* or *miss* from *this*. Other causes of damage to the inner ear include high fever or chronic illnesses, certain powerful medications, trauma to the head and genetic disorders. The auditory nerve can be damaged by abnormal growths (tumors) and other causes. See Chapter 4 for more detailed information about sensorineural hearing loss.

Mixed hearing loss

Some people may have a combination of both types of hearing loss. For example, someone with age-related hearing loss may develop an ear infection. The conductive part of the hearing loss caused by the infection can usually be eliminated with medical treatment, but not the sensorineural damage.

Central auditory processing disorders

Injury to the auditory processing centers of your brain — caused by trauma, disease or a genetic disorder — may occasionally cause hearing problems. These cases often are associated with problems of interpreting sound, such as locating its source, distinguishing between sounds, recognizing frequency patterns and listening to multiple sources at once.

Compensating for hearing loss

Hearing loss all too often bears the brunt of jokes and comedic skits. Inevitably it's associated with inattention, lower intelligence or "getting old." Some people simply resign themselves to not needing to hear everything out there anyway. But not being able to hear sufficiently can be an obstacle at best and dangerous at worst. Hearing not only helps you to understand others but also cues you to where you are and what is happening around you. Hearing keeps you socially and physically connected to the world.

Many people avoid admitting to a hearing loss for fear of being stereotyped as someone who consistently misunderstands conversation and interacts with others by shouting. They may compensate for their diminished hearing and try to mask it by:

- Asking others to repeat themselves
- Blaming others for mumbling or speaking too softly
- Limiting or withdrawing from social activities
- Turning up the volume on the television or radio
- Smiling and nodding without understanding

If you regularly engage in the actions listed above, you might consider seeking the help of an audiologist to evaluate your hearing. To deny a real hearing deficit because you don't want others to recognize it is like refusing to look at your shirt in order to detract attention from a stain. Many people will see through your efforts and notice the problem. Addressing your hearing problem can put you on the way to becoming a more active participant in life and a more engaged companion and friend.

Recognize signs of hearing loss

To get the most out of your hearing, look for early signs of hearing loss. The questions below, developed by the National Institute on Deafness and Other Communication Disorders, may help you decide whether to see a doctor or audiologist about a hearing evaluation. But remember that these are only general questions.

- Do you have a problem with hearing on the telephone?
- Do you have trouble following a conversation when two or more people are talking at the same time?
- Do people say that you turn the TV volume up too high?
- Do you have to strain to understand conversation?
- Do you have trouble hearing in a situation with a noisy background?
- Do you find yourself asking people to repeat themselves?
- Do many people you talk with seem to mumble or not speak clearly?
- Do you misunderstand what others are saying and respond inappropriately?
- Do you have trouble understanding the speech of women and children?
- Do people get annoyed because you misunderstand what they say?

If you answered yes to three or more of these questions, you may want to consider a hearing test. In addition, ask someone who knows you well to go through these questions with you in mind. He or she might notice signs of hearing loss in you long before you do and prompt you to get help.

Chapter 2

Getting a hearing exam

In the past year, perhaps you've noticed how much more difficult it has become to socialize with others. You're unable to hear
parts of words when someone is speaking to you. In conversation you miss shades of meaning and intention that everyone else
seems to pick up on. Because you're unsure of what's been said,
you're more reluctant to join in. If these situations seem familiar, a
hearing exam may help you identify a hearing problem and lead to
treatment that enables you to hear better and feel more involved
with others.

If you want to get your hearing or your child's hearing checked,
whom do you see? You might start by talking with your primary
physician or your child's pediatrician. Your doctor can do a preliminary exam of the ears and offer explanations for many of your
questions. He or she can also refer you to an appropriate hearing
specialist — an audiologist — if necessary. You can also consult an
audiologist directly.

In this chapter you'll get a closer look at each of the hearing specialty areas that may be involved at one point or another in the
diagnosis and treatment of hearing loss. You'll also find out when a
hearing exam may be necessary, what's involved in the exam and
what the results of the exam mean. Knowing what to expect can
help you get the most out of a hearing exam.

Who provides ear care?

Your family doctor may ask you from time to time about your hearing and encourage you to get a hearing test when appropriate. It's wise to contact your doctor whenever you're routinely exposed to loud noises or if you notice any signs of hearing loss. And see your doctor before attempting to buy a hearing aid. Sometimes hearing loss results from an infection, a tumor or another problem that calls for medication or surgery, not a hearing aid. Your doctor can guide you to the most appropriate treatment.

As you seek professional help, you may meet several kinds of hearing specialists, primarily otolaryngologists, otologists and audiologists. Because hearing loss may have a variety of causes, hearing specialists often work closely with specialists in other fields to determine the best course of treatment.

Otolaryngologists

Your family doctor may refer you to an otolaryngologist (oh-toh-lar-in-GOL-uh-jist) for a detailed examination of your ears. Otolaryngologists are medical doctors trained to diagnose and treat diseases of the ears, sinuses, mouth, throat, voice box (larynx) and other structures in the head and neck region. They also perform cosmetic and reconstructive surgery of the head and neck. These doctors are also known as otorhinolaryngologists (oh-toh-rye-no-lar-in-GOL-uh-jists) or ear, nose and throat (ENT) physicians.

All otolaryngologists have completed medical school and at least five years of residency, or specialty training. They're also certified by the American Board of Otolaryngology. After residency some otolaryngologists pursue an additional one or two year fellowship for more extensive training in a particular specialty.

Otologists

An otologist (oh-TOL-uh-jist) is an otolaryngologist who has completed a specialty fellowship focusing on ear disorders. Thus, he or she has the most training devoted to any physical problems of the ear. If your primary doctor suspects that you have a form of ear disease, you may be referred directly to an otologist. Some of the conditions that otologists treat include ear infections, facial paralysis, dizziness, hearing loss, ringing in the ears (tinnitus), tumors and congenital deformities. If you need surgery for an ear disorder, you'll probably see an otologist or an otolaryngologist with special training in ear surgery.

Audiologists

An audiologist (aw-de-OL-uh-jist) is trained to evaluate the perceptual aspects of your hearing. If you complain of hearing loss but your doctor finds no signs of ear disease, he or she may refer you to an audiologist. An audiologist can assess the type of hearing loss and measure its severity through various tests. Audiologists also evaluate and fit hearing aids and help with hearing rehabilitation.

Audiologists hold a master's degree or doctoral degree in audiology and must complete a year of fellowship training before practicing independently. They're certified by the American Speech-Language-Hearing Association (ASHA). Most states require audiologists to be licensed or registered in the state in which they practice.

Working together

Often, ear specialists work together to reach an appropriate diagnosis and pursue a form of treatment. For example, if you're about to receive treatment, your otologist may refer you to an audiologist so that your hearing can be measured before treatment, and again afterward. An audiologist who suspects, upon evaluation, that your hearing loss is due to a medical problem will refer you to an otologist or otolaryngologist for treatment. Subsequently, he or she may see you again for hearing rehabilitation. The proper sequence of visits to each specialist is important because each one is approaching the problem from a different perspective.

In some cases an audiologist monitors a person's hearing while he or she is undergoing treatment for an illness such as cancer or infectious disease. For example, some chemotherapy and antibiotic drugs can damage a person's hearing mechanism, so an oncologist or infectious disease specialist will work closely with an audiologist to monitor the person's hearing and ensure that the prescribed dosage is low enough to help avoid auditory damage.

Who should have a hearing exam?

People of all ages get hearing exams, from newborns to older adults. A hearing exam can be done when you request it or when a situation occurs that increases your risk of hearing loss. Sometimes an exam is mandated by law.

Children

The screening of newborns is now common practice in most hospitals in the United States. In many states it's mandatory. That's because each year more than 4,000 babies are born with a hearing impairment. Failure to identify the impairment early enough can lead to delayed speech and language development.

Children with unidentified hearing loss often don't do as well in school as their peers do. They're also more likely to be held back a grade or drop out. Because the loss of hearing isn't readily observable, adults often attribute a child's perceived inattention to other causes, such as laziness. Early intervention can help prevent many of the problems related to hearing loss and provide the child with tools necessary to reach his or her full potential.

Some types of hearing loss in children don't develop until months or years after birth, so periodic screening is recommended during the infant and toddler stages and throughout the school years. See pages 22 and 23 for the recommended screening schedules. In addition, babies considered to be at high risk of hearing loss should be screened regularly. This group includes infants with a medical history of:

- Severe oxygen deprivation at birth (birth asphyxia)
- Exposure in the womb to an infection such as German measles (rubella) or syphilis
- Exposure to herpes during passage through the birth canal
- An infection such as bacterial meningitis
- Severe jaundice
- Head trauma
- A nervous system disorder associated with hearing loss
- A chronic ear infection
- A family history of childhood hearing loss

Adults

Screening for adults is generally done at their request. ASHA recommends that adults get their hearing checked every 10 years through age 50 and every three years after that. Hearing loss increases with age — 30 percent of those age 65 or older and 14 percent of those between 45 and 64 years have hearing loss.

Employees

Prolonged exposure to high levels of noise is known to cause gradual, often permanent, hearing loss. The Occupational Safety and Health Administration (OSHA) requires that employers monitor their companies for noise levels at or above 85 decibels (db), averaged over eight working hours. Under such conditions the employer must develop and maintain a hearing conservation program at no cost to the employee. The program would include regular hearing (audiometric) testing, noise monitoring, access to earplugs or hearing protective devices (commonly known as earmuffs), record keeping and employee training regarding hearing protection (see "Recommended screening schedules").

If regular screening indicates that an employee is losing his or her hearing, the employee must be informed and must wear hearing protectors. In addition, hearing protectors are required when work noise levels exceed 90 db, if the levels are averaged over eight hours. In order for the hearing protectors to be effective, it's important that they fit properly and be worn continuously during noise exposure. OSHA also requires that an audiologist or an otolaryngologist or other qualified doctor administer the program.

What's involved in a hearing exam?

A doctor and an audiologist will complete different portions of the hearing examination in order to assess all aspects of your hearing. They will evaluate the signs and symptoms of your condition. They will also check for any other medical condition that may be causing the problem. This will help them to determine the severity of your hearing loss and suggest an appropriate course of treatment. The

Recommended screening schedules

Infants[1]

- Initial screening by 1 month of age, preferably at birth.
- If indicated by initial screening, further evaluation to confirm hearing loss by three months of age.
- Initiate appropriate treatment for infants with hearing loss before 6 months of age. Ongoing monitoring every three months.
- Screen children deemed to be at high risk of hearing loss every six months until age 3.

School-age children[2]

- On first entry into a school system.
- Annually from kindergarten through 3rd grade.
- At 7th grade.
- At 11th grade.
- On entry to special education.
- On repeating a grade.
- On entry to a new school system without evidence of previous screening.
- When indicated by a parent or caregiver, by a medical or school concern, or by high-risk factors of hearing loss.

tests will involve an overall medical evaluation that includes a medical history, physical examination of your ears and laboratory tests. Audiologic exams include audiometry, speech reception and word recognition, among others.

Medical evaluation
The first step in your hearing exam, whether you consult your family doctor or an ear specialist, is to get a full medical evaluation. This helps the doctor determine the overall status of your health and whether your hearing loss is the result of an underlying syn-

Adults[3]

- Every 10 years through age 50 and every three years thereafter.

Employees[4]

- Before employment.
- Before assignment to a hearing-hazardous work area.[5]
- Annually while assigned to a hearing-hazardous work area.
- After ending assignment to a hearing-hazardous work area.
- At termination of employment.

[1]Joint Committee on Infant Hearing Year 2000 Position Statement: Principles and Guidelines for Early Hearing Detection and Intervention Programs

[2]American Speech-Language-Hearing Association (ASHA)

[3]ASHA

[4]National Institute for Occupational Safety and Health

[5]A hearing-hazardous work area is considered an environment with noise exposure equal to or greater than 85 decibels, if averaged over eight hours.

drome or disease. The medical evaluation generally includes some or all of the following components:

Medical history. Your examiner will want to fully document the development of your hearing problem. He or she may ask questions such as:

- When did the signs and symptoms of hearing loss begin?
- Is the impairment in one ear or both ears?
- Is the problem getting worse, improving or staying the same?
- Are some sounds more difficult to hear than other sounds, or are all sounds equally hard to distinguish?

- Do you have difficulty recognizing where a sound comes from?
- Are you experiencing other signs and symptoms, such as ear pain, discharge, infection, dizziness, ringing in the ears and loss of balance?
- Do any members of your family have hearing problems?

Be sure to tell your examiner if you've had lengthy exposure to noise, either at work or home. In addition, tell him or her if you've ever had head trauma, ear surgery or a chronic illness, or whether you've recently had an upper respiratory infection, such as a cold or pneumonia. Let your examiner know what medications you're taking or have recently taken.

Physical exam. The next step will be to examine the size, shape and position of your outer ear (pinna) and to inspect it for any swelling, deformity or redness. This step may yield information about other problems that may be causing the hearing loss. Your examiner may check your eyes, nasal cavity, mouth and neck for any problems that might be associated with ear damage. A slender, flexible tube with a light at the end is used to check for signs of fluid buildup or infection in the back of your nose and upper throat (nasopharynx) and your eustachian tubes, which connect your ears to your nasopharynx.

Otoscopy. The examination of the ear canal, eardrum and middle ear is called an otoscopy. Your doctor or audiologist uses an instrument called an otoscope, which contains a light and magnifying lens. He or she may also use a specially designed microscope to

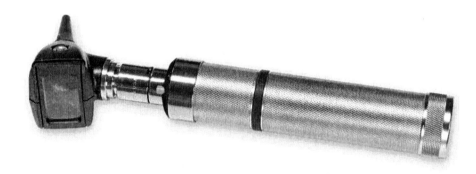

An otoscope is used to illuminate and magnify the inside of the ear, allowing the doctor to check for abnormalities.

view the ear canal and eardrum. Generally, an otoscopic examination is painless and takes a minute or two. Your doctor or audiologist may look for wax or fluid buildup, foreign objects, a tumor or skin abnormalities in the ear canal, and tears or perforations in the eardrum. He or she can also see whether the eardrum is translucent and has its normal pearly gray color. A bulging of the eardrum membrane may indicate a middle ear infection.

Tuning fork test. A preliminary hearing test using a tuning fork can be performed in your doctor's office. A tuning fork looks like a dining fork with only two tines. Made of steel, it sounds a single tone when struck against a solid object. To conduct the test, vibrating forks with different pitches are placed near your ear to measure your hearing sensitivity to air conduction of the sound wave. The forks are also placed against your head to measure your sensitivity to bone conduction of the sound wave.

People whose hearing is reduced by air conduction but is normal by bone conduction typically have conductive hearing loss — the sound wave has difficulty passing through the ear canal or the middle ear. People whose hearing is reduced both by air conduction and bone conduction generally have sensorineural hearing loss from damage to the inner ear.

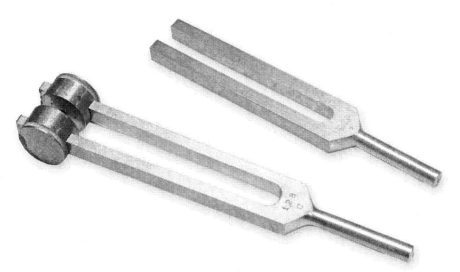

A tuning fork test may help determine if hearing loss is conductive (outer or middle ear problems) or sensorineural (damage to the inner ear).

Laboratory tests. Your examiner may request certain blood tests to confirm or rule out possible infectious or inflammatory diseases that are sometimes associated with hearing loss. These include syphilis, German measles (rubella), cytomegalovirus — a gastrointestinal infection — and autoimmune disorders. This type of test is particularly important for pregnant women. Such a disease in an expectant mother can lead to hearing loss that's present at birth (congenital) in her baby. Blood samples also may be looked at for DNA abnormalities.

Imaging tests. If your examiner suspects that a tumor, tissue abnormality or auditory nerve damage is the cause of your hearing loss, he or she may request detailed images of the interior of your head. Technology to produce these images includes magnetic resonance imaging (MRI) and computerized tomography (CT). Magnetic resonance imaging creates detailed images of soft tissues using magnetic fields and radio waves. Computerized tomography produces cross-sectional images of bone structures by using a computer to aggregate information from a series of X-rays. The images provide a glimpse of what would otherwise be unseen and can help your doctor diagnose a number of disorders. This type of imaging may also be used to locate congenital abnormalities, trauma-related damage and some tumors.

Audiologic exam

An audiologic exam is focused on hearing function — how well you hear. Audiologists use various tests to determine a person's hearing status and degree of hearing loss. These tests can help distinguish between different types of possible impairment, reveal whether an impairment is in one or both ears and determine whether the hearing loss involves one, two or more frequencies. Sequential or repeat testing can gauge whether the hearing loss is getting worse. Audiologic tests are usually conducted using electronic equipment in a room designed to muffle sound so that background noise doesn't interfere with the test.

Audiometry. A method of testing called audiometry measures your ability to hear pure tones, such as a middle C and higher notes, through air and through bone. The previously described tun-

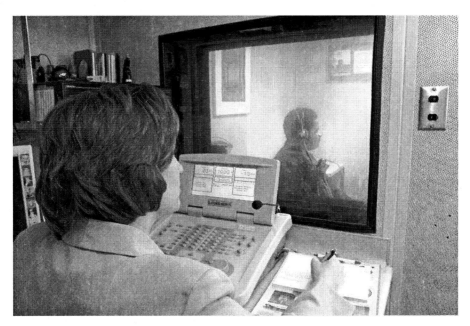

During audiometry, you'll be seated in a sound-treated room separate from the audiologist (front). You'll signal the audiologist whenever you hear a tone played through the earphones, and your responses will be recorded on an audiogram. This test determines the faintest sounds you can hear — known as hearing thresholds — which indicates your current degree of hearing loss.

ing fork test is a rudimentary form of the audiometric test. To check your hearing by way of air conduction, the audiologist begins by placing a pair of earphones over your ears or small, soft tips attached to earphones into your ear canals. He or she then introduces certain tones through the earphones to one ear at a time. By varying the frequency and intensity of the tones, the examiner can determine the faintest sounds you can hear (hearing thresholds). You'll be directed to signal the audiologist, usually by raising a hand or pressing a button, whenever you hear a tone. Your responses are recorded on a graph called an audiogram.

Checking your hearing for sounds conducted through the bones of your skull can help isolate problems in the outer and middle ear. To do this the audiologist places a special vibrating device either behind your ear or on your forehead. The vibrations travel through your skull, thus bypassing any blockage that may be present in the outer or middle ear. If test results show that you hear better when sound is conducted through the skull bone than through the air-filled passageways of your outer ear and middle ear, then sound isn't getting through the outer ear and middle ear properly. It's likely that you have some form of conductive hearing loss. If results show that your hearing is no better via bone conduction than through air conduction, it's likely to be a sensorineural problem with the inner ear.

Speech reception test. During a speech reception test, the audiologist speaks or plays a recording of two-syllable words, such as *pancake* or *baseball*, as you listen through headphones. Each syllable in a word is usually pronounced with an equal emphasis. As you hear a word, you repeat it or point to a picture of it. The sound of the words gradually becomes softer until you can no longer hear them. The faintest level of speech you can understand at least half the time is called your speech reception threshold.

Word recognition test. A word recognition test determines how well you can identify single-syllable words, such as *come* and *knees*. As the audiologist says the words or plays the words from a recording, at a constant, comfortable volume, you repeat each word or point to a picture of it. Your score reflects the percentage of words you identified correctly. The words may be spoken or played at a certain volume to determine how well you hear speech at normal conversational levels. Occasionally, background noise is added to see how distraction might affect your understanding. A word recognition test performed with and without a hearing aid can verify whether the device is improving your hearing.

Other tests

Along with giving you a medical evaluation and audiologic exam, your doctor or audiologist may wish to conduct other tests in order to study all aspects of your hearing. These tests can help to refine the diagnosis or determine which treatment options would be most beneficial. Some of these additional tests are:

Tympanometry. This test is used to check the function of your eardrum and middle ear. Tympanometry (tim-puh-NOM-uh-tre) can help detect problems such as a perforated eardrum, fluid in the middle ear and reduced air pressure in the middle ear resulting in a retraction of the eardrum.

Levels of hearing loss

Decibel (db) range	Level of hearing loss	Characteristics
16 to 25 db HL	Slight to minimal	• Has difficulty hearing faint or distant sounds
26 to 30 db HL	Mild	• Occasionally misses consonants • Has increasing difficulty in understanding with noisy backgrounds and faraway speakers
31 to 50 db HL	Moderate	• Can understand normal conversation if face to face and vocabulary is controlled
51 to 70 db HL	Moderate to severe	• May miss most of what's said in a normal conversation • Has difficulty listening in a group setting
71 to 90 db HL	Severe	• May not be able to hear speech unless very loud • Needs amplification to be able to converse normally
91 db HL and above	Profound	• May not be able to hear speech at all • Relies on visual cues such as lip reading or sign language

Source: American Speech-Language-Hearing Association, 2003

To conduct the test, your examiner places a soft probe in your ear canal. As small, varying amounts of air pressure are directed toward your ear, the device measures the corresponding movement of the eardrum. The results are charted on a graph called a tympanogram. Normal response produces a line rising to a sharp peak in the middle of the graph. But if fluid is in the middle ear, the eardrum doesn't move easily and the graph's line doesn't peak. The graph can also reveal whether the air pressure in the middle ear is less than or greater than atmospheric pressure.

Acoustic reflex test. An acoustic reflex test measures the sound level at which the muscles in the middle ear contract in response to sounds that are too loud (see page 12). During the test you hear a series of sounds at varying levels of intensity. The sound level at which an acoustic reflex contraction occurs, or the absence of any acoustic reflex, can help your examiner evaluate your hearing loss and locate problems along the auditory pathway.

Auditory brainstem response test. This test measures the electrical nerve impulses sent from the inner ear to the brain when sounds are heard. Electrodes are placed in the ear canal or near the ear as well as on the head. Earphones are used to introduce short clicking sounds to the ear. The electrodes record brain-wave activity on a graph as the auditory nerve receives the sound impulses and transmits them to the brain. Because this test doesn't require a voluntary response, such as a hand signal, from the person being tested, it's often used to screen hearing in newborns and infants. This test can be used to assess other problems with the auditory nerve.

Otoacoustic emissions test. This test measures an interesting phenomenon that occurs in the hair cells of the inner ear. As mentioned previously, these hair cells bend with the movement of fluid in the snail-shaped cochlea. The resulting vibrations of the hair cells produce inaudible sounds (echoes) called otoacoustic emissions. These emissions can be measured by placing a probe equipped with a microphone into the ear canal. This test is useful because people with normal hearing produce otoacoustic emissions, but people with hearing loss caused by damaged hair cells don't. This test is also used to screen hearing in newborns and infants because it doesn't require a voluntary response.

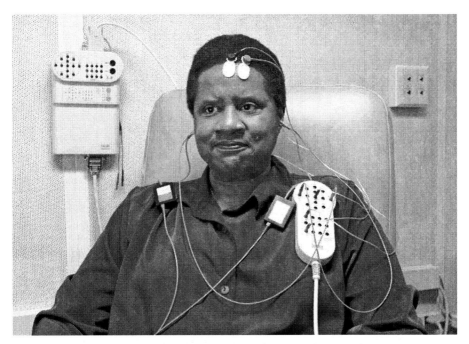

During an auditory brainstem response test, electrodes are attached to your ears and head to measure how the auditory nerve receives sounds and transmits them to the brain.

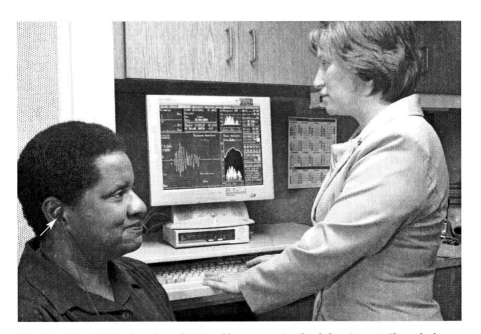

A probe with a small microphone is placed in your ear to check for otoacoustic emissions (arrow). These inaudible echoes aren't produced in people with hearing loss and thus do not register during the test.

Understanding your audiogram

Your doctor or audiologist may use any or all of the tests described in the previous section to compile a complete and detailed picture of your hearing. But the test that's relied on most often is the audiometric test. The resulting graph, the audiogram, provides an important overview of your hearing. In particular, the graph reveals your ability to hear the sounds of speech. At first glance an audiogram may seem pretty baffling (see below). To understand what the lines and numbers represent, it's helpful to look at each component of the graph separately.

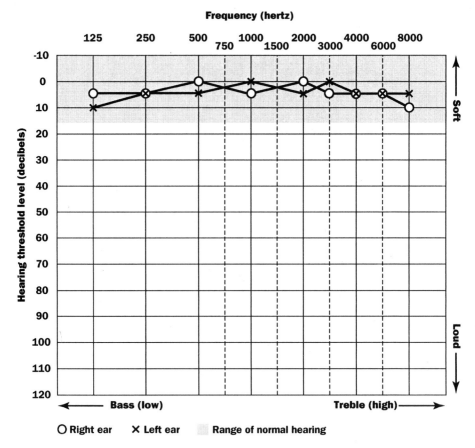

Audiogram showing normal hearing in the right ear and the left ear. Hearing in the right ear is plotted with Os and in the left ear with Xs. If your hearing is normal, all your Xs and Os will generally fall in the –10 decibels hearing level (db HL) to 15 db HL range. As hearing loss occurs, the Xs and Os fall lower and lower on the graph.

The audiogram portrays sound in terms of two of its most important qualities: frequency (pitch) in cycles per second, or hertz, and intensity (loudness) in decibels. The vertical lines represent a range of frequencies. This range moves from a bass or low pitch on the left (125 Hz) to a treble or high pitch on the right (8,000 Hz). Some speech sounds carry very low tones, such as the *vvv* in *vacuum* or the *mmm* in *morning*. Speech sounds such as *fff* as in *food* and *thh* as in *thanks* have a high pitch.

The horizontal lines on the audiogram represent how loud the sound is. These levels range from –10 db at the top of the graph (soft) to 120 db at the bottom (loud). Zero represents the very faint sounds that someone with normal hearing can generally hear.

Any point on the audiogram represents a sound at a certain pitch at a given level of loudness. When you take the audiometric test, your responses to different tones are recorded on the graph. At each frequency that's sounded, the faintest tone that you can hear in your left ear is recorded as an X and the faintest tone you can hear in your right ear is recorded as an O. The resulting lines of Xs and Os represent your hearing thresholds for your ears.

Some people may have symmetrical hearing loss, which means the loss is approximately at the same level in both ears. Others may have asymmetrical hearing loss, which means one ear hears better than the other. In addition, hearing loss may vary according to frequency. For example, someone may have normal hearing at low and middle frequencies in both ears. But he or she may have moderate to severe loss at high frequencies in the left ear and only mild loss at high frequencies in the right ear.

If you represented all of the sounds that make up human speech at a normal conversational level, you'd end up with a concave-shaped area just above the middle of the graph. It's called the speech spectrum (see page 34). Softer, high-pitched sounds such as *sss* and *thh* would be higher and toward the right within the spectrum. Louder, low-pitched sounds such as *mmm* and *ahh* would be lower and toward the left. Sounds such as *eee* fall in between.

If the speech spectrum were to be superimposed over your audiometric test results, you would be able to see which portions of conversational speech you can and can't hear.

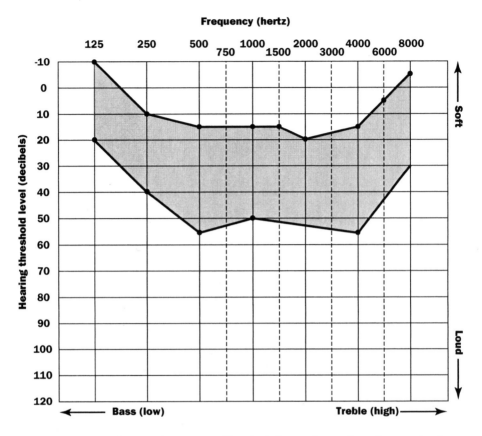

Audiogram showing the speech spectrum. The shaded area shows where the sounds of normal human speech lie in an irregular concave arc.

Taking action

Sometimes you don't think about getting your hearing checked until you notice that something is obviously wrong or another person calls a hearing problem to your attention. Hearing loss can be tough to admit to and is often viewed as a sign of old age.

But protecting or improving your hearing can have an immediate and positive impact on your quality of life — physically, socially and emotionally. Treatment can help eliminate feelings of isolation, shame and frustration. Better hearing can help you participate more actively in the world around you. A decision to take action and have a hearing exam can determine how well you'll hear weeks, months and years from today.

Chapter 3

Common problems of the outer ear and middle ear

A primary function of both the outer ear and the middle ear is to direct sound waves to the sensitive auditory structures of the inner ear. This conductive function allows strong, clear signals to be processed by the brain into sounds you can make sense of and recognize.

Conductive hearing loss occurs when something interferes with the passage of sound waves through the outer ear and middle ear. Very often, the function of the inner ear remains normal. When you have conductive hearing loss, all sounds that you hear, no matter the frequency (pitch) or level of intensity (loudness), seem to be muffled. What are soft or faint sounds to someone with normal hearing become inaudible to you.

A number of problems can obstruct the sound waves on their passage to the inner ear. The problems include too much earwax in your outer ear, a ruptured eardrum or an infection that causes a buildup of fluid in your middle ear.

Often, conductive hearing loss can be reversed with proper treatment, sometimes involving self-care and sometimes requiring medication or surgery. Problems of the outer ear and middle ear generally don't cause permanent damage. This chapter describes many of the common causes of conductive hearing loss and guidelines for the treatment of these conditions.

Outer ear problems

Problems that occur in your outer ear are more often a discomfort and annoyance than a serious medical condition. With proper self-care and, if necessary, treatment from a doctor, outer ear problems usually can be resolved and your hearing restored to its former level. The most common outer ear problems include earwax blockage, foreign object lodged in the ear and swimmer's ear.

Earwax blockage

Skin lining the outer portion of your ear canal contains glands that produce a waxy substance called cerumen, more commonly known as earwax. This wax is part of your body's normal defense against harm. It traps dust and other foreign particles in the outer ear to keep them from injuring the more delicate eardrum (tympanic membrane). Wax also helps inhibit the growth of bacteria.

Normally, earwax migrates to the external edge of your ear canal and either falls away or is wiped away when you clean your outer ear. But at times you may produce more wax than your ear can expel, causing the wax to accumulate in your ear canal.

Generally, excessive earwax doesn't lead to hearing loss because it doesn't completely block the passageway. But many people insert objects such as cotton swabs, hairpins, keys and even a finger into the ear canal, presumably to clean it. This action can push the wax farther into the passageway and impact it. Impacted earwax can reduce your hearing by blocking airborne sound vibrations in your ear canal. Blockage can also give you an earache and cause tinnitus (noise such as ringing, buzzing or roaring in your ears). You may feel as if your ear is full or plugged.

Treatment. To remove excess wax from your ears, you may wish to consult a doctor or you may try the following self-care method:
- Soften the earwax with a few drops of baby oil, mineral oil or olive oil from an eyedropper twice a day for several days.
- When the wax is softened, fill a bowl with water heated to body temperature — if the water is colder or hotter than body temperature, application may make you feel dizzy during the procedure.

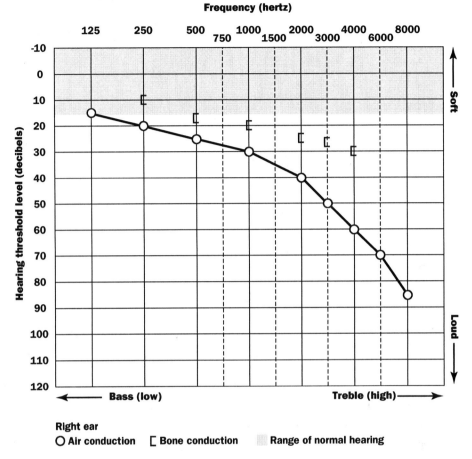

Frequency (hertz)

Right ear
O Air conduction   [Bone conduction   ▒ Range of normal hearing

A typical audiogram of hearing loss due to earwax blockage in the right ear. Results show increasing difficulty in hearing sounds at higher frequencies. You would need sounds at 6,000 hertz to be at least 70 decibels HL in order to hear them.

- With your head upright, grasp the top of your ear and pull upward. With your other hand, squirt water gently into your ear canal with a 3-ounce rubber bulb syringe. Then lower your head to the side and allow the water to drain into the bowl.
- You may need to repeat the previous step several times before the excess wax falls out.
- Dry your outer ear carefully with a towel or hand-held hair dryer. Inserting a few drops of an alcohol-vinegar preparation (half rubbing alcohol, half white vinegar) with an eyedropper also will help dry your ear.

Earwax removers sold in stores (Murine, others) also can be effective. One note of caution: If you've previously ruptured an eardrum or had ear surgery, don't flush your ears unless your doctor approves. Such action could lead to infection.

If after self-care you still have excess wax in your ears, it may be best to seek the help of your doctor. He or she may repeat the washing of your ears or use special instruments to either scoop or suction out the wax.

Foreign object in the ear

Occasionally, an object such as a piece of cotton thread from a swab, a bit of paper, an earplug or even an insect can become stuck in your ear. You may notice this when your ear begins to tickle, hurt or feel plugged. Most foreign objects lodge in the ear canal and don't cause lasting hearing problems. But if an object becomes lodged or is pushed too far into your ear, it may rupture your eardrum and potentially damage your middle ear, which can have more serious consequences.

Treatment. Here's some advice for occasions when an object becomes lodged in the ear:

- Don't attempt to remove the foreign object by probing with a cotton swab, matchstick or any other tool. To do so is to risk pushing the object farther into the ear, making it harder to extract and possibly causing more serious damage.
- You may be able to dislodge the object by tilting your head toward the affected side and shaking it gently in the direction of the ground.
- If the object is clearly visible to an observer, is pliable and can be grasped easily with tweezers, he or she may be able to gently remove it.
- If the object isn't readily accessible, contact your doctor or a hospital emergency room. A doctor may remove the object by using tiny forceps or suction or by flooding it out with fluid. He or she can check to see if any damage has occured.
- If an insect is lodged in the ear and is still alive, tilt the affected ear upward. Insects instinctively crawl up, rather than down, in order to free themselves.

- If the insect doesn't exit the ear on its own, place a few drops of warm — not hot — baby oil, mineral oil or olive oil into the ear. You can ease the entry of the oil by gently pulling the top of the pinna back and upward. The insect should suffocate and float out in the oil bath.
- Don't use oil to remove objects other than an insect. Also, don't apply oil if any of the signs or symptoms of a perforated eardrum are present, such as pain, bleeding or discharge from the ear.

Swimmer's ear

Swimmer's ear (otitis externa) is an infection of the ear canal. It's the result of persistent moisture in the ear — for example, from frequent swimming — often in combination with a mild injury to skin in the ear canal. Such an injury can result from scraping the ear canal when trying to clean out wax. These are ideal conditions for bacteria and fungi to invade the tissue of the ear canal and cause an infection. Hair spray and hair dyes also may cause infection. Swimmer's ear is most common in young adults.

Pain or itching in the ear, a swollen ear canal and the drainage of pus are signs and symptoms of an outer ear infection. Temporary hearing loss may occur if swelling or pus blocks the ear canal.

Treatment. If the pain is mild and you don't have ear drainage or hearing loss, follow the self-care tips below. Otherwise, seek medical attention.

- Place a warm — not hot — heating pad over your ear. But don't lie on the heating pad.
- Consider taking a pain reliever such as ibuprofen (Advil, Motrin, others) if needed.
- Keep water and other substances out of your ear canal while it's healing.
- Place a few drops of an alcohol-vinegar preparation (half rubbing alcohol, half white vinegar) in your ear after showering or swimming. The alcohol helps dry the skin of the ear canal, and the vinegar helps prevent bacterial and fungal growth.

Over-the-counter ear-water drying drops also are available for use after swimming (Auro-Dri, Swim-Ear, others).

If the ear pain doesn't subside or you have additional concerns, see your doctor. After cleaning your ear, your doctor may prescribe eardrops containing a corticosteroid to relieve itching and decrease inflammation, and antibiotics to control the infection. More severe infections may be treated with oral antibiotics.

In a few instances, particularly among people with diabetes or a weakened immune system, swimmer's ear may lead to infection of the bones and cartilage at the base of the skull (malignant otitis externa). Such a complication can be life-threatening and usually requires prolonged antibiotic therapy under the care of a team of specialists, such as an otologist, endocrinologist and infectious disease specialist.

Eardrum problems

As resilient as your eardrum (tympanic membrane) is, its fragile structure is subject to constant use and constant strain. Two common problems are a ruptured eardrum and barotrauma. Both conditions can result in hearing loss mostly caused by a disruption or distortion of the eardrum, which prevents it from vibrating properly in response to sound waves. Usually, the hearing loss is slight and temporary.

Ruptured eardrum
Your eardrum is a thin, delicate membrane that plays the crucial role of gatekeeper for sound waves traveling from your outer ear to your middle ear. The eardrum may be torn or perforated as a result of an ear infection or trauma to the ear.

Ear infection. Fluid buildup in the middle ear caused by an infection can exert undue pressure on the eardrum and force it to rupture. Pain associated with the buildup usually resolves itself once the eardrum has ruptured, relieving the pressure as fluid drains out of the ear. Chronic ear infections also can wear down the eardrum and create a perforation on its surface.

Trauma to the ear. The eardrum can be ruptured by a sharp blow to the head or increased air pressure from outside, such as

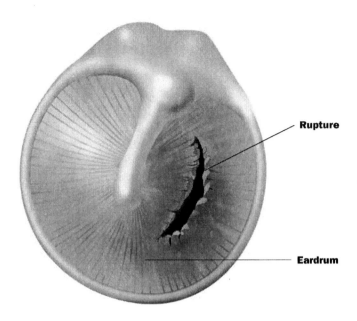

Rupture

Eardrum

Although a ruptured eardrum usually will heal itself, the risk of infection and hearing loss still exists. It's important to see your doctor if you think your eardrum may be damaged.

that caused by an explosion, a slap across the ear or a diving accident. The eardrum can be punctured if you push an object such as a cotton swab or paper clip too far into the ear canal.

Signs and symptoms of a ruptured eardrum include earache, partial hearing loss, tinnitus (noise such as ringing, buzzing or roaring in your ears) and slight bleeding or discharge from the ear. In some cases the ossicles in the middle ear also may be damaged, resulting in more severe hearing loss.

Treatment. Usually, a ruptured eardrum heals by itself without complications and with little or no permanent hearing loss. Large ruptures may cause recurring infections. If you think you may have a ruptured eardrum, see your doctor right away. Meanwhile, these self-care tips may ease ear pain and promote healing.

- Take aspirin or other pain reliever if needed.
- Place a warm — not hot — heating pad over your ear.
- Keep your ear dry.
- Before showering place into the ear canal a cotton ball coated with petroleum jelly to keep water out.

Your doctor may prescribe an antibiotic to prevent infection in the middle ear. He or she may also place a thin paper patch over your eardrum to seal the opening while it heals. If your eardrum hasn't healed within three months, you may require a surgical procedure to repair the tear.

Barotrauma

Barotrauma (bar-oh-TRAW-muh), also called airplane ear, results from a disparity between air pressure in the atmosphere and air pressure in your middle ear. Normally, the eustachian tube, a narrow channel that connects your middle ear to the back of your nose and upper throat, allows air to flow in and out of your middle ear when you swallow or yawn. This movement of air helps maintain equal pressure on both sides of your eardrum.

Barotrauma may occur when you experience a sudden and drastic change in atmospheric air pressure, such as a rapid descent during an airplane landing or a rapid ascent from a deep-sea dive. Another way barotrauma can develop is when the eustachian tube becomes blocked or fails to deliver air properly to the middle ear. This may happen when you have a congested nose from a nasal allergy, cold or throat infection.

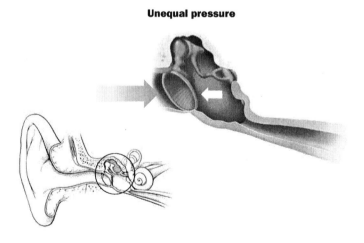

Barotrauma commonly occurs in situations such as flying or scuba diving, when you experience a sudden change in air pressure. Your ears may feel plugged or painful because the air pressure in your middle ear is lower than the air pressure in the atmosphere.

Either situation — a rapid change in atmospheric pressure or restricted airflow in the eustachian tube — can lead to lower air pressure in your middle ear than in the atmosphere. This causes your eardrum to move inward (retract). The distortion of your eardrum interferes with the passage of sound waves, so your hearing is slightly reduced.

Activities that involve rapid changes in external air pressure may require you to open your mouth or swallow frequently to equalize the air pressure in your ears. The signs and symptoms of barotrauma include pain in one or both ears, slight hearing loss and a feeling that both ears are plugged.

A more serious problem may occur if the air pressure change is extreme or if your eustachian tube is completely blocked. The small blood vessels in your middle ear may rupture and bleed, filling your ear with blood and resulting in hearing loss.

Treatment. Although barotrauma may cause discomfort, it's not a serious condition and doesn't result in permanent hearing loss. The pain usually disappears within a few hours after it begins, and hearing returns to normal.

If you're going to fly or scuba dive with a congested nose, try taking a decongestant (Afrin, Neo-Synephrine, others) one hour before the activity. This will help prevent blockage of your eustachian tubes. During a flight, suck candy or chew gum to encourage swallowing. A method used by pilots and divers is to pinch the nostrils shut, inhale and swallow. The pop in your ears is a sign that air has gone through the eustachian tube to your middle ear.

If your symptoms persist, consider seeing your doctor. On occasion it's necessary to make a small incision in your eardrum to equalize air pressure and remove fluid from your middle ear, a procedure known as myringotomy (mir-ing-GOT-o-me).

Middle ear problems

A variety of problems, such as infections, cysts, tumors and abnormal bone growth, can affect your middle ear. These problems are frequently associated with hearing loss caused by a disturbance of either the eardrum or the tiny bones in the middle ear: the hammer (malleus), anvil (incus) and stirrup (stapes). Often, hearing can be restored with medical or surgical treatment. However, if the problem extends to the inner ear, permanent hearing loss may occur.

Middle ear infection

An inflammation or infection of the middle ear is known as otitis media. It's usually associated with a cold, sore throat or other respiratory infection that blocks the eustachian tube. The blocked tube prevents the middle ear from being properly ventilated, causing the inflammation and an accumulation of fluids such as pus and mucus. In addition, bacteria in the nose, mouth or throat may travel through the lining of the eustachian tube and infect the middle ear. Acute otitis media is a single, severe episode that typically lasts no more than three weeks.

With a middle ear infection, fluid often accumulates in the middle ear to the point where it obstructs the movement of the eardrum and the ossicles, causing conductive hearing loss. If too much fluid accumulates, the eardrum may rupture. As the ear infection gets worse, it usually causes a painful earache. Other signs and symptoms that may be associated with ear infection include dizziness, loss of balance, nausea, vomiting, ear drainage and fever. At times, pus and mucus may persist in the middle ear even after the infection has passed, causing recurring episodes of infection and persistent hearing loss (see "Chronic ear infection").

Although otitis media may occur at any age, it's most common in young children. This is partly due to the shape and orientation of a child's eustachian tube, which is shorter and more horizontal than an adult's. A more horizontal orientation means fluid is less likely to drain and more likely to accumulate in a child's ear. The fluid itself isn't necessarily a problem. But it's an ideal breeding ground for bacteria or viruses that cause infection.

Treatment. The pain, fever or drainage so often associated with a middle ear infection will more than likely cause you to see a doctor. If you have an infection, the doctor's examination of your ear may reveal a red, bulging or indented eardrum. Tympanometry, a type of hearing test, will indicate reduced pressure in the middle

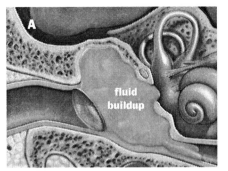
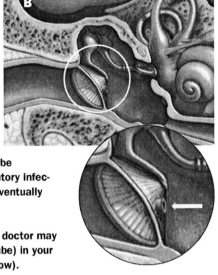

(A) Otitis media may occur if the eustachian tube becomes blocked due to a cold or other respiratory infection. Fluid may build up in the middle ear and eventually become infected.

(B) To treat chronic middle ear infections, your doctor may place a temporary drainage tube (ventilation tube) in your eardrum to relieve pressure and drain fluid (arrow).

ear or diminished mobility of the eardrum. If fluid is draining from your ear, your doctor may take a sample of the fluid and send it to a laboratory to identify the organism that's causing the infection.

Your doctor will likely prescribe antibiotics to clear up the infection in your ear. After the infection is gone, the fluid usually disappears within three to six weeks. Once you begin taking the antibiotics, it's important to complete the full prescription even if your symptoms improve. This ensures that all of the bacteria are killed.

Your doctor may also prescribe decongestants if nasal congestion is contributing to your ear infection. Hearing tests are typically administered to monitor your improvement.

Chronic ear infection

Chronic otitis media is a recurring or persistent middle ear infection. It may occur as a complication of an acute case of otitis media. Sometimes, a low-level infection continues even after treatment has been undertaken to eliminate it. In other cases, the initial acute infection clears up after treatment, but the ear is left more vulnerable to future infections.

The signs and symptoms of chronic ear infection are often milder than those of an acute infection, but in the long run they can be more dangerous. If the eustachian tube is consistently blocked, the tissues of the middle ear gradually thicken and become inflamed. The mucus they secrete also thickens. A vacuum created in the middle ear by the blocked tube can deform or rupture the eardrum. As these changes come about, the structures of the middle and inner ear slowly deteriorate, causing permanent damage and hearing impairment. Infection can also spread to the bone behind the ear — a projection of bone called the mastoid process — and even to the brain.

If pus begins to seep from your ear canal and your ear hurts or you notice hearing loss, it would be best to schedule an appointment with your doctor as soon as possible. He or she can have an audiologist perform hearing tests to determine the type of hearing loss and the degree of severity. The doctor will also examine your ear to identify the source of infection. A computerized tomography (CT) scan of your head may be used to see if infection has spread to the mastoid process.

Treatment. Your doctor may try to treat the cause of eustachian tube blockage, such as a cold or allergies, in order to improve airflow to your middle ear. If an active bacterial infection is present, antibiotic therapy is typically prescribed. The medication may be taken orally or by way of eardrops. If the medication is effective, you should start feeling better in a few days. If the middle ear remains filled with fluid and the eardrum is still intact, a small surgical incision in your eardrum may be necessary to relieve pressure and help drain fluid. The incision in the membrane usually heals in about a week, sometimes before all of the fluid has drained out. To prevent this, your doctor may temporarily place a tiny ventilation tube in the incision to ensure complete drainage (see the illustration of otitis media on page 45).

If significant damage has been done to the eardrum and ossicles, more extensive surgery may be needed to remove infected tissue and repair these structures. This procedure is known as tympanomastoidectomy (tim-puh-no-mas-toid-EK-tuh-me). The surgery may be done all at once, or the infection may be eliminated first and the middle ear structures reconstructed during a later surgery. Individuals with chronic ear infections often need multiple surgeries. Hearing should improve as the ear heals.

Cholesteatoma

A cholesteatoma (ko-le-ste-uh-TOH-muh) is the growth of normal skin tissue in the wrong place. It often occurs when skin from the ear canal grows through a hole in the eardrum and extends into the cavity of the middle ear. It may also happen when a blocked eustachian tube creates a vacuum in the middle ear, drawing the membrane of the eardrum inward to form a pocket. Old skin cells that are caught in the eardrum pocket contribute to the formation of a cholesteatoma.

Occasionally, during fetal development, skin cells become trapped behind the eardrum so that a baby is born with congenital cholesteatoma. This type of cholesteatoma may grow quickly.

Some of the signs and symptoms of a cholesteatoma include pus drainage from your ear, hearing loss, ear pain or numbness, headache, dizziness and weakness of your facial muscles. The degree of hearing loss depends on where the tissue grows. Frequently, it encroaches on the ossicles, impeding the sound vibrations and causing significant conductive hearing loss.

The development of a cholesteatoma can erode bone, which makes this a potentially serious condition. It may invade the mastoid bone behind your ear. If left untreated, a cholesteatoma will continue to grow and may eventually destroy the bony structures of not only the middle ear but also the inner ear, damaging the cochlea and the vestibular labyrinth. This results in sensorineural hearing loss and problems with balance. Uncontrolled growth of the cholesteatoma can also damage the facial nerve. In severe cases it may penetrate the brain, causing an infection of the brain.

Treatment. A cholesteatoma is removed surgically. If the growth is very small, your doctor may remove it in a single operation. A larger or more advanced cholesteatoma may require a series of operations to correct damage to the bones of your middle ear and possibly to rebuild them. If all of the growth isn't removed, it will grow back, possibly requiring operations at a later time.

In severe cases, where the cholesteatoma has affected your mastoid bone, your doctor may perform a radical mastoidectomy (mastoid-EK-tuh-me). This leaves a cavity that can be cleaned out periodically, but doesn't restore damaged bones or lost hearing. In a

modified radical mastoidectomy, the surgeon attempts to recon-
struct the ossicular bones with an artificial replacement (prosthesis)
or cartilage. This may help preserve or improve hearing.

Other cysts and tumors

Other abnormal growths may develop in the middle ear or sur-
rounding tissues, such as the temporal bone of the skull, although
these types of growths are less common. Most middle ear tumors
are noncancerous (benign), although some, such as squamous cell
carcinoma, are cancerous (malignant) and capable of spreading to
other parts of the body. Benign tumors usually grow slowly, whereas malignant tumors tend to grow at a faster rate.

A sensation of the affected ear being plugged may indicate a
tumor. So can hearing loss or tinnitus (noise such as ringing,
buzzing or roaring in your ears), drainage from the ear, facial paralysis, dizziness and loss of balance. If you experience any of these
symptoms, plan to see your doctor. A CT scan or magnetic resonance imaging (MRI) can help determine if a tumor is present. If
that's the case, your doctor may take sample tissue from the tumor
for analysis to determine whether it's malignant.

The more common tumors include:

Glomus tympanicum and glomus jugulare. Both of these
tumors are masses of cells than can grow in the middle ear and
interfere with vibration of the ossicles, leading to significant hearing loss. Often a glomus tumor will cause a pulsing sound in your
ear that accompanies each heartbeat. Most glomus tumors are
benign, although in rare instances they can spread to the lymph
nodes in your neck and become a more serious problem.

Squamous cell carcinoma. Malignant tumors of the ear are rare.
Of those that do occur, squamous cell carcinoma (SKWAY-mus sel
kahr-sih-NO-muh) is the most common. This type of tumor usually
develops in skin cells of your pinna and ear canal or in your middle
ear and mastoid. Though what causes the tumor is unclear, it has
been associated with chronic inflammation of the ear. Ear pain,
periodic draining of fluid from the ear and extended periods of
bleeding from the ear are signs and symptoms of squamous cell
carcinoma. This cancer is usually fatal if left untreated.

Tumors of the ear are usually surgically removed. The surgery is delicate and complex and may involve removing some or all parts of the ear, depending on the nature and size of the tumor. This can result in permanent loss of hearing, as well as loss of function in the nerves leading to your face and shoulder. Radiation therapy may be used as a primary treatment or in combination with surgery to improve the chances of survival. With malignant tumors, radiation therapy is often used after surgery to destroy any remaining cancerous cells.

Otosclerosis

Otosclerosis (oh-toh-skluh-ROH-sis) develops when an abnormal growth of spongy bone forms at the entrance to the inner ear (oval window). Due to this growth, the stirrup, one of the tiny bones in the middle ear, gradually becomes fixed to the oval window and loses its ability to vibrate. In some cases, the cochlea of the inner ear becomes involved, causing greater hearing loss.

Otosclerosis is the most frequent cause of middle ear hearing loss in young adults. It's twice as common in women as in men and affects whites more often than people of other races. Signs and symptoms usually appear between the ages of 15 and 35. The development of the disease is slow, and it can affect one or both ears. In women with otosclerosis, the rate of hearing loss may increase during pregnancy.

An increasing amount of evidence suggests that genetic defects may predispose a person to the disease — around half those individuals with otosclerosis have a family history of the disease. Other recent studies indicate that the measles virus may be a factor in the development of otosclerosis.

Treatment. Because otosclerosis typically results in a mild to moderate hearing loss and progresses little beyond that, hearing aids can successfully overcome most hearing loss that has occurred.

Another option is surgery to remove the fixed stirrup from the ear and insert a tiny wire or prosthesis made of platinum, titanium, teflon or stainless steel. This procedure is known as a stapedotomy (sta-puh-DOT-uh-mee). The prosthesis can help most people with otosclerosis, but in a few cases it may cause total loss of hearing.

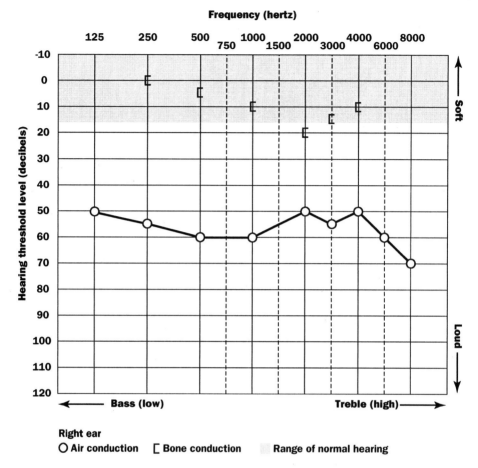

A typical audiogram of hearing loss due to otosclerosis in the right ear. Because the stirrup can no longer vibrate to transmit sound waves to the inner ear, air conduction for all frequencies is much less than normal.

The prosthesis may also become displaced, a growth of spongy bone may recur over the oval window, or the anvil (incus), to which the prosthesis is attached, may erode. If the disease continues to progress after surgery, the ability of the prosthesis to function may be greatly reduced.

If you have otosclerosis, you may be told to take tablets of sodium fluoride, but the value of this treatment is debated. The rationale for this treatment is that fluoride may help the spongy bone to harden, preventing progressive changes in the inner ear and the resulting hearing loss. Another form of medical treatment that's

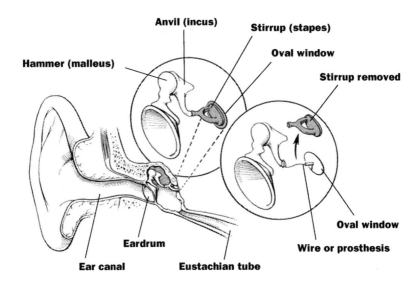

Anvil (incus)
Stirrup (stapes)
Oval window
Hammer (malleus)
Stirrup removed
Oval window
Eardrum
Wire or prosthesis
Ear canal
Eustachian tube

In a stapedotomy, the malfunctioning stirrup (stapes) of the middle ear is replaced with a tiny wire or prosthesis that transmits sound vibrations to the inner ear.

being investigated is the use of bisphosphonates, a class of drugs typically prescribed for osteoporosis. Bisphosphonates inhibit the breakdown of bone that occurs in the normal cycle that bone undergoes to keep itself healthy.

Ossicular chain disruption

A traumatic head injury can result in the displacement or breaking (fracture) of the small bones of the middle ear. These bones — the hammer, anvil and stirrup — are referred to as the ossicular chain. The most common site of displacement from a trauma is at the joint where the anvil connects to the stirrup. Frequently, the anvil itself is partially broken. The disruption of the ossicular chain causes a breakdown in the passage of sound waves from the eardrum to the inner ear, resulting in significant hearing loss.

Treatment. Obviously, a complete medical examination should follow any serious head trauma. Hearing tests can help determine the nature of any hearing loss and the degree of its severity. If you still have hearing loss six months after the trauma, your doctor may propose surgery or recommend that you talk to an audiologist about a hearing aid to remedy your loss.

Surgery involves a procedure called ossiculoplasty (o-SIK-yoo-loh-plas-te), which attempts to rebuild the displaced ossicles or to replace them either with a prosthesis or with small pieces of bone or cartilage. Because the ossicles are so small, the operation is a delicate one, and you may not recover all of your hearing. If the head trauma has caused damage to the cochlea, resulting in sensorineural hearing loss, a hearing aid may be the best option, as surgery won't rectify the cochlear damage.

Although complications are rare, some of the risks that accompany all types of ear surgery are:

- Total deafness in the affected ear
- Tinnitus
- Dizziness and loss of balance
- Damage to the facial nerve resulting in changes to your sense of taste or facial paralysis on the affected side

Your ear doctor will discuss such risks with you before any decision is made regarding surgery.

Chapter 4

Common problems of the inner ear

The word *sensorineural* refers to the response of cells to stimuli from the outside environment and the internal workings of the body. With regard to hearing, it involves receptor cells in the cochlea, the primary structure of the inner ear, and the auditory nerve that links the inner ear to the brain.

The organ of Corti, located inside the cochlea, contains rows of ultrasensitive receptors known as hair cells, which respond to the incoming stimuli. These hair cells convert sound waves into electrical impulses that are carried by the auditory nerve to information processing centers in the brain.

Sensorineural (sen-suh-re-NOOR-ul) hearing loss involves damage to the inner ear, the auditory nerve or the brain. For example, when some of the hair cells of the organ of Corti are damaged or other changes take place in the cochlea or to the auditory nerve, the electrical impulses aren't transmitted as efficiently, resulting in a loss of hearing.

The most common form of sensorineural hearing loss is that associated with aging. It's known as presbycusis (pres-bih-KU-sis). As you get older, the hair cells within your cochlea gradually wear out, causing you to lose sensitivity to sound. Some adults may lose very little hearing as they age, whereas others lose considerably more due to hair cell loss.

Noise is another cause of sensorineural hearing loss because it can damage your inner ear. It's likely that for many older adults, hearing loss is due to a combination of aging and noise exposure over the years. Other causes of sensorineural hearing loss are disease, trauma and genetic disorders.

Unfortunately, sensorineural damage is often permanent, and the hearing loss is irreversible. But with the use of hearing aids and other assistive hearing devices and techniques, it's still possible to communicate effectively, even with a hearing impairment.

Presbycusis

Presbycusis refers to age-related hearing loss. It's well-known that as people age, their hearing tends to decrease. Around 30 percent of Americans who are age 65 and older have hearing loss, whereas only about 3 percent of those under 45 have hearing loss, according to a survey conducted for the Centers for Disease Control and Prevention and the National Center for Health Statistics.

Because there's so much variation in how people grow old, the effects of aging on the human body are hard to describe precisely. In general, though, you can expect that as you age, physical and mental changes will cause your senses to become a little less sharp and sensory details a little harder to distinguish. In your ears, for example, you may lose some of the hair cells in your cochlea. This is probably the most common cause of sensorineural hearing loss. In addition, nerves may become a little slower at transmitting messages to and from the brain, and your brain may not be as quick to interpret sounds.

Initially, you may lose sensitivity to sounds with a higher frequency (pitch). This is because damage to the hair cells often occurs first at a location where high-frequency sounds are generally processed. When this happens, you may be unable to hear or distinguish between sounds of speech that have a high frequency, such as *sss*, *fff* and *thh*. At the same time, your ability to hear sounds with a low frequency may remain intact. Some sounds, such as a booming bass instrument or a passing truck, may even seem too loud.

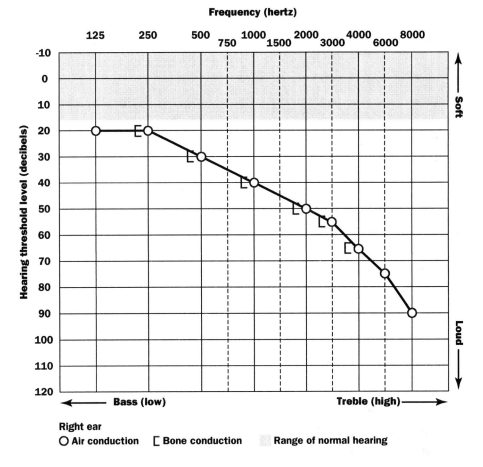

Frequency (hertz)

Right ear
○ Air conduction   ⊏ Bone conduction   ▓ Range of normal hearing

Audiogram of the right ear showing a typical pattern of hearing loss due to presbycusis. Often as you age, your sensitivity to low-frequency sounds remains intact but you'll have increasing difficulty hearing high-frequency sounds. Many high-frequency sounds, such as doorbells or bird songs, may become inaudible.

Presbycusis is sometimes accompanied by ringing or buzzing in your ears, a condition known as tinnitus (TIN-ih-tus). Presbycusis also makes it hard to hold a conversation in an area with background noise, such as a busy store. Not being able to hear everything in a conversation is like reading only parts of a story or overhearing music from a passing car outside while you're indoors. It's usually a frustrating, if not annoying, experience.

Presbycusis tends to run in families, which means genetics is likely involved. The onset of hearing loss can be earlier in some families than in others. Aside from genetics, other factors that may compound age-related sensorineural hearing loss include:

- **Noise.** The cumulative effect of a lifetime of noise, such as the sounds of power tools, machinery, appliances, firearms and loud music, can gradually affect your ability to hear.
- **Medications.** Some drugs are harmful to your hearing mechanism and are said to be ototoxic (oh-toh-TOK-sik).

Just as you can make adjustments for other changes that accompany aging, you can compensate for hearing loss. In particular, hearing aids can make high-frequency sounds audible without amplifying low-frequency sounds that you can already hear.

Noise-induced hearing loss

Every day we're surrounded by noise — traffic sounds, the hums and grinds of appliances, people conversing, the music and chatter from radio and television, airplanes flying overhead. Typically we think nothing of noises like this. Most of the time they aren't loud enough to annoy us or hurt our ears. But sometimes a noise is too loud for our ears to handle. Some sounds can cause permanent damage. The two primary ways that noise can damage hearing are a sudden explosion of noise and prolonged exposure to loud noise:

- **Sudden explosion of noise.** A one-time unprotected exposure to sound measuring 140 db or above, such as a rifle gunshot, can cause immediate hearing loss. The sounds of artillery and machine guns are even worse. In fact, noise-induced hearing loss is the most common injury in the U.S. Army. Firecrackers in close hearing range also can damage your hearing.
- **Prolonged exposure to loud noise.** Regular exposure to noise levels above 85 db can, over time, damage your hearing. This can happen at work or during recreational activities. Sources of loud noise include power tools such as chain saws, power lawn equipment, tractors, combines, motorcycles, snowmobiles and sound equipment set to a high volume.

If you experience hearing loss due to a sudden exposure to loud noise, you'll probably notice it right away. With prolonged expo-

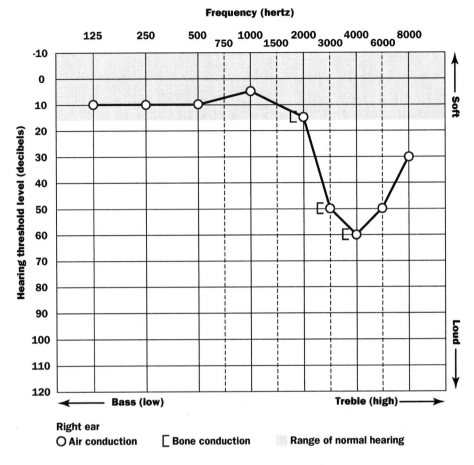

Audiogram of the right ear showing a typical pattern of hearing loss due to noise. Hearing sounds at low frequencies may remain in the normal range, while the ability to hear high frequencies takes a characteristic dip, greatest at 4,000 hertz.

sure to noise, the hearing loss may be so gradual and painless that you may not notice a problem until someone else brings it to your attention or you're informed of the results of a hearing test. Noise-induced hearing loss may occur in one or both ears and is often accompanied by the ringing or buzzing in your ears known as tinnitus, which may or may not subside.

If your hearing loss is temporary, it's called a temporary threshold shift. With this condition, normal hearing usually returns within 16 hours of being exposed to the noise. In other cases, hearing loss resulting from exposure to loud noise may be permanent.

Approximate sound levels of common noises

Sound level (decibels)	Noise
30	Whisper
60	Normal conversation
80	Ringing telephone
90	Hair dryer, power lawn mower
98	Hand drill
105	Bulldozer
110	Chain saw
120	Ambulance siren
140	Jet engine at takeoff
165	12-gauge shotgun blast

Source: National Institute for Occupational Safety and Health, Centers for Disease Control and Prevention, 2001

Although noise-induced hearing loss can't be restored, it can be prevented. If you can't avoid the loud noise, wear hearing protective devices (earmuffs) or earplugs when involved in loud activities. So how loud is too loud? Here's a good rule of thumb: If you have to shout in order to be heard by someone an arm's length away, you're exposed to too much noise.

Hearing protectors are effective when they're worn for 100 percent of the time you're exposed to loud noise. Whatever type of ear protection you use, make sure it's clean and fits you correctly. Earplugs should maintain an airtight seal in your ear. Earmuffs must contact the skin entirely around your ear. Commercially made ear protectors that meet federal standards are available at drugstores, hardware stores and sporting goods stores. Earplugs and earmuffs can reduce noise by about 15 to 30 decibels. When worn together, they offer an additional 5-db noise reduction.

In companies that operate at noise levels averaging 85 db over an eight-hour day, employers are required to have a hearing conservation program, which includes conventional noise measurements, provision of hearing protectors, an annual hearing test to screen employees, record keeping, and employee education and training. See Chapter 2 for information on hearing screening. If testing reveals significant hearing loss in an employee, he or she is required to wear hearing protectors. If noise levels reach 90 db or above, everyone is required by law to wear hearing protectors.

Sudden deafness

Sometimes hearing can be lost all at once or within only a few days. This condition is known as sudden sensorineural hearing loss (SSNHL). You may notice a popping sound when it happens, or you may detect it when you first wake up or try to use the impaired ear. SSNHL is almost always confined to one ear. Dizziness or tinnitus also may accompany this type of hearing loss. About 4,000 cases of sudden deafness occur every year in the United States. It's most common in young or middle-age adults.

Sudden deafness is a medical emergency. As soon as you notice it, contact your doctor immediately. You'll be given a hearing test to determine the extent of your hearing loss. The less hearing loss that has occurred, the more likely that hearing may return to normal within a couple of weeks. Although many individuals with SSNHL regain their former level of hearing, some may experience no recovery or regain only partial hearing in the affected ear.

Pinpointing the cause of SSNHL can be a difficult task. If your hearing returns quickly, you may not need medical treatment. If the cause is known, addressing the underlying problem may resolve the hearing loss. When the cause isn't obvious, your doctor may consider several possible suspects, including:
• A viral inner ear infection
• An abrupt disruption of blood flow to the cochlea
• A tear in a membrane within the cochlea
• An acoustic neuroma

Most of the time the cause is unknown. In such a case, your doctor may prescribe a corticosteroid such as prednisone or dexamethasone to reduce inflammation and help your body fight disease. Or he or she may prescribe an antiviral medication such as acyclovir.

Hold down the noise

Most of us understand the dangers of work-related noise. But we easily overlook the racket at home. Here are steps you can take to keep down the noise level around the house:

- Turn down the volume on your television or stereo.
- Choose personal stereos with an automatic volume limiter.
- Don't turn up the volume on headphones to drown out background noise. Try earplugs instead.
- Choose quieter appliances.
- Place pads under noisy appliances.
- Don't run multiple appliances at the same time.
- Install carpeting to absorb sound.
- Seal windows and doors to block the noise of traffic.
- Wear earplugs or earmuffs when using power equipment.
- Rest your ears. Alternate noisy activities with quiet ones.

Hearing loss that results from recreational activities is becoming more common. Don't forget to wear ear protectors when riding a snowmobile or motorcycle, shooting a gun or listening to extremely loud music.

Other causes of hearing loss

Aging and noise are the most common causes of sensorineural hearing loss, but a number of other factors may damage the inner ear and auditory nerve. The hearing loss may be sudden or may worsen gradually.

Viral infections

Before widespread immunization against measles and the mumps, the viruses that cause these illnesses were also major causes of hearing loss in children. The measles virus usually attacks cells lining the lungs and the back of the throat. The mumps typically affects the parotid glands — one of three types of salivary glands — between the ear and the jaw. From these areas of the head, either infection may spread to your inner ear and destroy hair cells and nerve endings in the cochlea. Viruses may also travel through your bloodstream to the cochlea. Other viral illnesses, such as influenza, chickenpox and mononucleosis, also may lead to hearing loss.

Hearing loss resulting from measles and the mumps is now rare in the United States because the infections can be prevented with a measles-mumps-rubella (MMR) vaccine. Children routinely get this shot at ages 12 to 15 months and again at three to six years. You also gain immunity if you've previously had a measles or mumps infection. If you're not sure whether you've been immunized or if you need a vaccination before traveling to a place where the illnesses are still prevalent, talk to your doctor about the vaccine.

Head trauma

Injury to your head can sometimes cause a hearing impairment, especially if the part of the skull above your ear (temporal bone) is fractured. Such a fracture may damage the delicate structure of the cochlea or the eighth cranial nerve, which consists of your auditory and vestibular nerves twined together. Damage to this nerve interferes with impulses being relayed to the brain. In some cases, hearing loss isn't apparent until some time after the trauma.

Normally, your brain rests inside your skull enveloped by spinal fluid. A sharp blow to your head will cause your brain to shift, which can lead to torn blood vessels, pulled nerve fibers and bruised brain tissue. Pressure waves from the blow can disrupt structures and fluids in the cochlea (cochlear concussion) and cause sensorineural hearing loss. If you've experienced a cochlear concussion, your hearing may improve over a six-month period. Another result of head trauma may be bleeding into the fluids of the cochlea, which also can result in hearing loss.

Trauma to your head may sometimes rupture the membrane covering the oval window between the middle ear and inner ear (perilymph fistula). This allows leakage of fluid into the middle ear and can lead to a hearing impairment.

Meniere's disease

Meniere's (men-e-AYRZ) disease is characterized by periodic attacks of dizziness, hearing loss, tinnitus and the feeling of a plugged ear. An attack may last anywhere from 20 minutes to two days. Typically, dizziness is the worst part and may make you feel nauseated. Attacks can occur daily or once a year. Between attacks you don't feel any symptoms. Although your hearing comes and goes with the attacks, it may gradually become worse. Meniere's disease usually affects only one ear.

No one knows what causes Meniere's disease, but scientists associate the signs and symptoms with a fluctuation in the volume of fluids in the inner ear. Excess fluid can increase pressure on, distort and occasionally rupture the membranes of your inner ear. This disrupts your sense of balance and your sense of hearing.

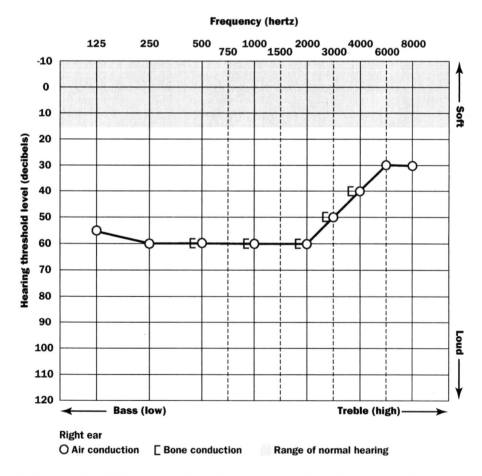

Right ear
O Air conduction   [Bone conduction   Range of normal hearing

Audiogram of the right ear showing how Meniere's disease typically affects hearing. During attacks, sounds at lower and middle frequencies are more difficult to hear than sounds at higher frequencies.

Treatment for Meniere's disease usually consists of taking medications to manage the symptoms of dizziness and nausea, limiting your intake of caffeine, alcohol and chocolate, and eating a low-salt diet. Limiting your salt intake can help decrease fluid levels in your body, including your inner ear, and possibly decrease the frequency of attacks. Your doctor may also prescribe a diuretic, antihistamine or migraine medication to help reduce fluid retention. If dizziness is so severe that it inhibits your daily life, inner ear surgery may be an option. For more information on surgery of this kind, see the brief summary on page 170.

Labyrinthitis
Labyrinthitis (lab-uh-rin-THI-tis) is an inflammation of the inner ear that affects the cochlea, which is vital to hearing, and the vestibular labyrinth, which plays a role in balance and eye movement. If the inflammation affects only the vestibular labyrinth, it's known as vestibular neuronitis. The exact cause of the inflammation isn't known, but it often follows a bacterial ear infection or a viral upper respiratory illness. It may occur after a blow to the head, or it may occur with no associated illness or trauma.

Signs and symptoms of labyrinthitis include dizziness, hearing loss, tinnitus, nausea, vomiting and involuntary movements of your eyes. You may lose all of your hearing in the affected ear.

To keep the condition from getting worse, it's helpful to sit still as often as possible and avoid sudden changes in position. Most of the time, the inflammation goes away on its own after a few weeks. If the underlying problem is bacterial, your doctor will likely prescribe antibiotics to get rid of the infectious agent. Your doctor may also recommend medications to relieve dizziness and nausea. If you receive prompt treatment, complications are rare.

Acoustic neuroma
An acoustic neuroma (vestibular schwannoma) is a slow-growing, benign tumor on the auditory and vestibular nerves. The tumor develops as a result of overproduction of the cells that cover and insulate the nerves. It's usually located at the point where the nerves exit the bony canal and enter the brain cavity.

Because an acoustic neuroma affects both the auditory and vestibular nerves, hearing loss in one ear, tinnitus and dizziness are common signs and symptoms of the disorder. As the tumor grows, it can affect other nerves, causing facial numbness and weakness.

Although an acoustic neuroma generally grows slowly, it can become large enough to push against the brain and interfere with life-sustaining functions. It's usually removed surgically, but it may also be treated with radiation therapy.

To remove an acoustic neuroma, the surgeon will make an incision behind or above your ear and remove a segment of your skull about the size of a silver dollar to get at the tumor. Once the tumor is removed, the bony segment or a permanent acrylic patch is used to cover the opening in the skull to help prevent infection and protect the brain. If the tumor can be removed without injuring the auditory nerve, your hearing might be preserved. This is possible if the tumor is small. In general, the larger the tumor, the greater are the chances of your hearing and facial nerves being affected.

A treatment to shrink or stabilize small or medium-sized tumors is gamma-knife radiation. This closed-skull procedure involves a

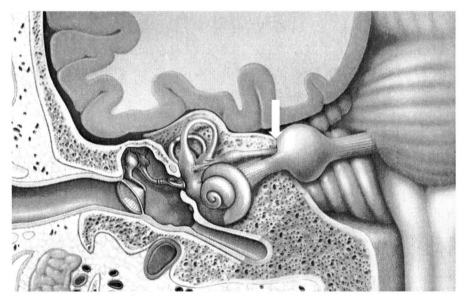

An acoustic neuroma is a tumor on the eighth cranial nerve, which consists of your auditory and vestibular nerves twined together. It generally develops at the point where the nerves enter the brain cavity (arrow).

machine that treats the tumors with highly focused radiation beams. One of the benefits of gamma-knife radiation is that the skull isn't opened, reducing the chances for infection. Another is that recovery time is shorter than that for surgery. A serious drawback is that it offers less certainty of long-term tumor control.

Reactions to medications

The action of certain medications or chemicals can cause hearing loss, tinnitus and balance problems. Medications can also aggravate an existing inner ear or hearing problem. These medications are considered ototoxic. The effects of ototoxic medications, which can range from mild to severe, usually depend on the dose and the length of time you take them, as well as factors such as heredity. Some ototoxic medications are listed on pages 66 and 67.

Hearing problems caused by some ototoxic drugs go away when you stop taking the medication. Drugs that are known to cause permanent hearing loss are usually given only when no other alternative exists for treating a life-threatening disease.

About 200 drugs are considered ototoxic. If you and your doctor decide that it's in your best interest to take an ototoxic drug, an audiologist will likely test your hearing before, during and after administration of the drug. The hearing test before you take the drug provides baseline information with which to compare later tests. While you're taking the drug, your physician will closely monitor test results to help decide how long you can continue or when to alter the dosage. If needed, the audiologist can help you plan for a hearing aid and hearing rehabilitation.

If you have existing hearing or balance problems or if you experience inner ear problems with certain medications, be sure to let your doctor know. Doing so can help you avoid unnecessary exposure to ototoxic drugs. Signs and symptoms of an ototoxic reaction to medication include:

- Onset of tinnitus
- Worsening of existing tinnitus
- A feeling that one or both ears are plugged
- A loss of hearing or worsening of existing hearing loss
- Dizziness, sometimes accompanied by nausea

Ototoxic medications

Listed below are some of the drugs that may cause hearing loss. If you're taking one of these medications, it's important not to stop taking it until you've consulted your doctor.

Class of drugs	Examples	Effects
Salicylates	• Aspirin • Aspirin-containing products	Ototoxicity usually occurs at high doses. Hearing loss is almost always reversible.
Quinine	• Chloroquine (Aralen) • Quinidine (Cardioquin) • Quinine (Quinamm) • Tonic water	Ototoxicity usually occurs at high doses. Hearing improves when use of the drug is stopped.
Loop diuretics (a specific type of water pill)	• Bumetanide (Bumex) • Ethacrynic acid (Edecrin) • Furosemide (Lasix) • Torsemide (Demadex)	Ototoxicity is temporary. If these drugs are given with an ototoxic antibiotic, risk of permanent damage may increase.

Autoimmune inner ear disease

Autoimmune inner ear disease (AIED) occurs when your body's immune system mistakes normal cells in your inner ear for a virus or bacteria and begins attacking them. This produces an inflammatory reaction in your inner ear and can lead to problems with both hearing and balance. AIED is rare, probably accounting for less than 1 percent of all cases of hearing loss.

Why your immune cells attack other normal cells is unclear. As with many other disorders, scientists suspect that AIED may have something to do with faulty genetics.

Class of drugs	Examples	Effects
Amino-glycoside antibiotics	• Amikacin (Amikin) • Gentamicin (Garamycin) • Neomycin (Mycifradin) • Streptomycin • Tobramycin (Nebcin) • Vancomycin (Vancocin)	Risk of ototoxicity usually increases when the antibiotic is administered directly into the bloodstream, which allows the greatest amount of the drug into the body. Damage may be permanent.
Anticancer drugs (antineoplastics)	• Carboplatin (Paraplatin) • Cisplatin (Platinol)	Drugs designed to kill cancer cells also may kill inner ear cells. The damage is often permanent and may make you more vulnerable to noise-induced hearing loss.
Environmental chemicals	• Lead • Manganese • n-Butyl alcohol • Toluene	Excessive exposure to these chemicals in the workplace may result in permanent hearing loss.

Signs and symptoms of AIED include hearing loss that usually begins in one ear and moves to the other, tinnitus, a feeling that an ear is plugged and, in about half the AIED cases, dizziness. Because these signs and symptoms are similar to those of other ear disorders, diagnosis can be difficult. In addition, AIED is often associated with other autoimmune disorders of the body, such as:

• Ankylosing spondylitis, a disease that affects your spine
• Sjögren's syndrome, also known as dry eye syndrome
• Cogan's syndrome, which affects your eyes and ears
• Ulcerative colitis, which affects your intestinal tract

- Wegener's granulomatosis, which inflames blood vessels
- Rheumatoid arthritis, which inflames your joints
- Scleroderma, which hardens and scars your skin and other connective tissues
- Systemic lupus erythematosus (SLE) and Behcet's syndrome, both of which can affect multiple systems in your body

If you have AIED, your doctor may prescribe corticosteroids (prednisone, dexamethasone) to reduce the inflammation. Corticosteroids have side effects that can limit their long-term use.

Other options are immunosuppressive agents such as cyclophosphamide (Cytoxan) and methotrexate (Folex, Rheumatrex). These drugs suppress your immune cells or prevent them from multiplying, but they can also damage other normal cells.

Plasmapheresis (plaz-muh-fuh-RE-sis) is a procedure that withdraws a certain amount of your blood, mechanically removes the offending antibodies and returns clean blood to your body. This can be an expensive procedure and must be done repeatedly.

Etanercept (Enbrel), an injectable drug used to treat other autoimmune diseases, may be of benefit to people with AIED. It works by blocking a naturally occurring protein (tumor necrosis factor) that, at elevated levels, may be to blame for the inflammation of autoimmune disorders.

If AIED has caused you to lose your hearing completely, then a cochlear implant may be an option for you.

Congenital hearing problems

A congenital problem means the condition exists at birth. These types of hearing problems can be hereditary in nature, or they may develop in the womb or during the birthing process.

It's estimated that genetic factors are responsible for more than 50 percent of all incidents of congenital hearing loss. A child whose hearing loss may be inherited usually has parents who each carry a recessive gene for hearing loss (autosomal recessive hearing loss). This gene isn't expressed in the parents, who have normal hearing, but is expressed in a child who inherits both recessive genes. So far, more than 15 genes have been identified that cause recessive hearing loss not related to any other illness.

Often, congenital hearing loss is part of a collection of symptoms (syndrome) caused by a genetic defect, such as:
- Down syndrome
- Usher's syndrome
- Treacher Collins syndrome
- Crouzon's disease
- Alport's syndrome

Congenital hearing problems are typically sensorineural. Factors that may cause hearing loss in an infant include:
- An infection that's present in the mother, such as German measles (rubella), cytomegalovirus, herpes or syphilis
- Premature birth
- A lack of oxygen during or shortly after birth
- Blood incompatibilities between the mother and child
- Diabetes in the mother
- Fetal alcohol syndrome
- Abnormal development of ear, face or neck structures

Most newborns are screened for hearing loss before they leave the hospital. It's important to continue monitoring your child's hearing, because a hearing impairment that goes unnoticed will significantly interfere with speech and language development, socialization and learning.

Research on the horizon

The fact that so much sensorineural damage causes permanent hearing loss has challenged scientists to come up with new approaches to treatment. They're testing certain drugs that may reduce the effects of loud noise exposure on the inner ear. And they're studying drugs that may be used to inhibit the effects of aging on your hearing.

Hair cell regeneration

An exciting area of new research involves hair cell regeneration. Hair cells are the delicate sensory receptors of the inner ear. Damage to the hair cells results in serious hearing problems.

Until the mid-1980s, scientists believed the inner ear was incapable of producing new hair cells. Then they discovered that birds have a natural ability to generate new hair cells in response to damage. The new cells restored the birds' hearing. This remarkable discovery has led researchers to study how to make regeneration happen in humans.

Research efforts have successfully induced the first stage of hair cell regeneration in the inner ears of mammals such as guinea pigs, rats and mice. Human hair cells might be stimulated to regenerate using hormone-like substances called growth factors, which control cell growth. Researchers are testing various growth factors to see which ones might cause hair cells to develop.

Scientists hope that one day they may be able to restore lost or damaged hair cells in humans in order to treat hearing and balance disorders. Although progress so far is promising, many challenges remain. Researchers must not only identify the substances that will cause regeneration but also find a workable method of delivering these substances to the inner ear.

Gene therapy

Scientists have also made dramatic progress in understanding the relationship between genetics and hearing loss. They've discovered that many genes play a role and that genetics and environment likely interact to influence hearing loss. For example, an individual may be genetically predisposed to hearing loss caused by specific environmental factors such as noise, drugs or illness.

With this body of knowledge, researchers are investigating gene therapy as a way to treat deafness. Gene therapy, also called gene transfer, involves replacing a defective gene with a normal gene in a specific cell and hoping that the cell will use it.

Gene therapy holds great potential for use in treating hereditary forms of deafness, preventing hair cell damage and stimulating hair cell regeneration. This research is still at an early stage, and there's a long way to go before an affordable, accessible genetic treatment for hearing impairment is feasible.

Chapter 5

Tinnitus

Tinnitus (TIN-ih-tus) is commonly described as sound in your ear that comes from no apparent source in your surroundings. The sound can be ringing, buzzing, whistling, chirping, hissing, roaring or clicking, among others. Some people even describe it as music or as the sound of boiling water. Often the noise seems to originate in your head. In some parts of the United States the word can also be pronounced tih-NI-tus.

Many people experience brief episodes of tinnitus after hearing a loud noise or taking certain medications, such as aspirin. Few people are alarmed by such episodes, and the noise goes away.

Persistent tinnitus is a common and usually benign condition. An estimated 40 million to 50 million adults in the United States experience it to some degree. Many don't find it bothersome.

Approximately 8 million to 12 million Americans are bothered by persistent tinnitus, some more severely than others are. They might describe their tinnitus as annoying and even debilitating. At night the ringing or hissing noise can make it difficult to fall asleep. Tinnitus can also make it hard for them to concentrate on a particular task. Frustration with the unexplained sounds can lead to anxiety, fear and depression. Tinnitus is also frequently associated with most other ear disorders as well as with other diseases, including cardiovascular disease, allergies and anemia.

Unraveling a mystery

Medical experts sometimes grapple with a precise definition of tinnitus. One reason is that it's unclear whether tinnitus is a syndrome — a set of symptoms that accompanies another, separate disorder — or whether it's a disorder in itself. The mechanisms that trigger tinnitus within the ear — explaining how and why the noise occurs — are unknown. Although descriptions of tinnitus exist as far back as the time of the Pharaohs of ancient Egypt, much about the condition remains a mystery.

Several theories have been proposed regarding what causes tinnitus. One hypothesis is that it's a phenomenon of the central nervous system, similar to the phantom-like sensations experienced after a limb amputation. A person may feel a pain in his or her foot even after that leg has been removed. In similar fashion, the central nervous system is somehow responding to hair cells that have been lost by stimulating electric signals to the brain.

Another theory suggests the disorder is centered in the brain. The evidence is based on positron emission tomography (PET) scans. PET scans reveal information about which part of the brain is being used to process information or to accomplish a specific task. Careful study of PET imagery of people with tinnitus suggests that tinnitus sounds stimulate a part of the brain different from that stimulated by external sounds.

Some researchers speculate that tinnitus arises in the cochlea, specifically from disorganized activity of the hair cells. Others think the cause may lie with the activity of chemicals in the auditory nerve, which carries messages between your inner ear and brain. Evidence also suggests that spontaneous nerve activity in the auditory pathway may be the culprit.

Regardless of their preferred theory, most scientists agree that multiple causes and mechanisms are probably involved in the development of tinnitus. Unfortunately for those with a condition that's persistent and bothersome, this lack of knowledge has often left them with no recourse but to live with the discomfort. The good news is that tinnitus is usually not a serious medical problem. In a few cases, tinnitus may be caused by an underlying condition

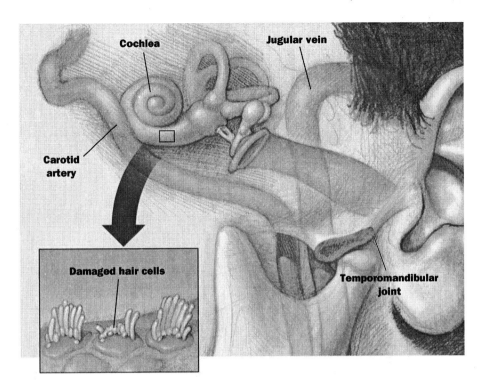

Cochlea

Jugular vein

Carotid artery

Damaged hair cells

Temporomandibular joint

Multiple causes are probably involved in the development of tinnitus. Some researchers think that tinnitus results from damage to the hair cells inside your cochlea. Turbulent blood flow through veins and arteries in the body also may produce a sound sensation. Blood vessels such as the carotid artery and the jugular vein lie close to the inner ear. Tinnitus may also result from a misalignment of the jaw joint (temporomandibular joint), which can produce a clicking or grating sound.

that's treatable. More often there's no cure, but you can learn various ways to manage tinnitus so that its effect on your daily life is minimized. These options often require the assistance of a doctor and audiologist along with your active participation.

Types

How people describe their tinnitus varies greatly from one person to the next. The only thing in common seems to be the existence of unexplained noise in their ears. To provide a general classification, some experts describe tinnitus as two broadly defined types: objective and subjective.

Objective tinnitus

Objective tinnitus, sometimes referred to as pulsatile (PUL-suh-tile) tinnitus, is a sound sensation that can be heard by other people as well as by you. The sounds originate within your body, most commonly from turbulent blood flow caused by blood vessel problems.

If you have atherosclerosis, for example, a buildup of cholesterol and other fatty deposits causes major blood vessels — including those in your neck and head — to lose some of their elasticity. This impedes the vessels from flexing or expanding slightly with each heartbeat. Narrower openings in the blood vessels require a more forceful blood flow. Your heart works harder, to a point where your ears can detect each heartbeat. Your doctor may hear the sound by placing a stethoscope on your head or neck.

High blood pressure and factors that may temporarily increase blood pressure, such as stress, alcohol and caffeine, can make the tinnitus even more noticeable. Repositioning your head usually can cause the sounds to disappear.

The malformation of small blood vessels (capillaries) connecting your arteries and veins also can produce an audible pulse. Other possible sources of objective tinnitus include muscle spasms, movement of the eustachian tube and spontaneous vibrations of the hair cells in your inner ear.

About 4 percent of the individuals with tinnitus have the objective type. Treating the underlying vascular disorder may help reduce or even eliminate the sounds. That's why it's important to describe the tinnitus to your doctor and get an accurate diagnosis. You can help your doctor by being as specific as possible about the noises you hear and under what circumstances they occur.

Subjective tinnitus

Subjective tinnitus involves sounds that only you can detect. Scientists aren't sure what causes these sounds and in order to study the problem must depend on how well people describe what they're hearing. In fact, some experts have compared the effort of defining subjective tinnitus to the popular fable of four blind men attempting to describe an elephant by touching it. Their consensus may in fact turn out to be quite different from the reality. But many

Hyperacusis

Hyperacusis (hi-pur-uh-KOO-sis) is another condition that's often associated with tinnitus. Hyperacusis involves an extreme sensitivity to sound. Everyday noise, such as traffic, conversation or telephone rings, seems uncomfortably loud. Like tinnitus, the cause of hyperacusis is unclear.

Hyperacusis may be even more debilitating than the tinnitus. A person with severe hyperacusis may avoid social situations for fear of painful noise exposure (phonophobia), choosing instead to stay in a secluded environment with little or no noise. Although some form of hyperacusis may occur in people with hearing loss, those reporting hyperacusis usually have normal hearing.

Treatment consists of managing the symptoms through counseling and participating in a program that gradually increases your tolerance of normal sounds. This may involve a white noise generator, an electronic device that generates a hissing sound similar to what you may hear when a radio is tuned between stations. Initially the device is tuned to barely audible levels and then gradually increased to higher levels for regularly set periods of time.

believe the problem originates somewhere within the structures of the inner ear, such as the cochlea and the auditory nerve, or within the auditory centers of the brain.

Although the precise nature of subjective tinnitus is unclear, several known factors may trigger the condition or make it worse:

Hearing loss. Exposure to loud noise can damage hair cells in your cochlea, causing permanent hearing loss. About 90 percent of people with tinnitus have some form of noise-induced hearing loss. It may be that the damage to hair cells also causes the tinnitus. Age-related hearing loss may precipitate tinnitus, as well.

In addition, as hearing loss muffles sounds from the outside world, your tinnitus may become more noticeable. Other conditions that can reduce your hearing, such as impacted earwax or an ear infection, also may increase tinnitus.

Medications. Over 200 prescription drugs are associated with tinnitus. Some of these are toxic and may permanently injure the ear. Usually they're prescribed only when absolutely necessary. Others can produce tinnitus and temporary hearing loss as side effects. Always discuss with your doctor the potential side effects of any prescription medication you're taking. After you begin taking the drug, let your doctor know if your hearing is reduced or you begin experiencing tinnitus. Stopping or adjusting the dosage of the drug can usually eliminate the tinnitus. If you already have tinnitus, tell your doctor. An alternative drug may be available.

Jaw disorders. A misalignment of the joint connecting your jaw and the temporal bone of your skull may result in clicking or grating noises whenever you move your jaw. Some claim the noises are present even when no jaw movement occurs, but this is debated. A dentist who specializes in treatment of this joint may be able to correct the misalignment and eliminate the associated noises.

Other factors. Various other conditions or circumstances are associated with tinnitus.

- Schwannomas (shwah-NO-muhz), which are benign tumors that grow on nerve fibers of the brain
- Trauma or injury to the head or neck
- Perilymph fistula, a rupture in the membrane covering the oval window (see page 172)
- Otosclerosis, or stiffening of the bones in the middle ear
- Meniere's disease, which causes excess fluid in the inner ear
- Exposure to excessive noise
- Excessive sodium intake in your diet
- Stress, either emotional or physical

Diagnosis

There's little doubt that tinnitus can drive some people to distraction. In many cases tinnitus creates a cycle of ever greater discomfort: The annoyance leads to increased attention to the noise, which results in more frustration. Some people find the distraction so severe that they're unable to carry on with regular activities.

Several options are available that will allow you to manage tinnitus so that you can function in a reasonable degree of comfort. First, talk about the condition with your doctor or audiologist. He or she can help rule out any treatable causes of your tinnitus. Other specialists may become involved in your diagnosis.

If your tinnitus is the result of an underlying condition, such as a tumor or circulatory disorder, medical or surgical treatment may resolve the problem. Measures such as treating an ear infection or removing impacted wax also may help reduce tinnitus.

If the cause remains unknown, you and your medical team can decide how best to treat your symptoms. A thorough medical history, physical examination, hearing tests and laboratory tests may all provide vital pieces of information. To get a more detailed picture of your tinnitus, your doctor may ask:

- Is one ear affected, or both? If only one, which one?
- Do you have hearing loss?
- What does the noise sound like? Is it high pitched or low pitched? How loud is it?
- Are the sounds constant, or do they change in loudness or change in pitch?
- What circumstances make the tinnitus better or worse?
- How does this condition affect your work, your sleep and your ability to concentrate?
- How has this condition affected your stress level?

Your audiologist may also try to determine the frequency (pitch) and intensity (loudness) of your tinnitus through audiologic tests. All of this information can help you and your medical team select a treatment that's best for your situation.

Management

Though many questions remain open about the cause of tinnitus and how the condition develops, treatment strategies focus on managing its signs and symptoms. This focus allows a person to continue functioning effectively in his or her daily responsibilities and to lead a more fulfilled life.

Management can range from using a hearing aid or masker — or a combination of both — to counseling and cognitive therapy. You and your medical team may try several approaches before deciding on the one that works best for you. Sometimes it's helpful to use multiple strategies to manage tinnitus.

Hearing aids and maskers
Treatment involving hearing aids and maskers attempts to include enough background noise into your hearing so as to cover over, or mask, the sounds of tinnitus. One way to do this, especially for people with hearing loss, is to wear a hearing aid. A hearing aid amplifies external sounds so that the tinnitus may seem less noticeable. If you don't have hearing loss, or if your tinnitus is at a different frequency from the hearing you've lost, a hearing aid may not be as helpful in reducing the annoyance of tinnitus. Hearing aids are discussed in greater detail in Chapter 7.

Another way to obscure tinnitus is by wearing a simple masker device that fits behind or in your ear. The device resembles a hearing aid, but instead of amplifying external sounds, it produces low-level background noise that's typically easier to tolerate than tinnitus. You can control the loudness of the masker. Its frequency is usually programmed by the manufacturer and your audiologist to achieve the best effect.

Another option is a device that's a combination hearing aid and masker. The device amplifies environmental sounds and speech but can also provide background noise to mask the tinnitus.

Sometimes tinnitus is most noticeable and bothersome at night, when the rest of the world is quiet. Some people use a bedside masker (loudspeaker) that allows them to select sounds, such as ocean waves, falling rain and white noise, as they prepare for bed. This type of masker can help them relax and obscure their tinnitus during periods of sleep or rest.

To the relief of some people with tinnitus, masking can sometimes produce what's called residual inhibition. This is a period of time when your perception of tinnitus is partially or completely reduced after removing the masker. These episodes may last from less than 30 seconds to two or three hours.

In certain situations, for example when someone with tinnitus also has total or nearly total hearing loss, the use of a cochlear implant may decrease tinnitus. A cochlear implant is a hearing device implanted behind the ear that picks up external sounds and sends them to the brain as electrical signals. These signals help the wearer hear speech and environmental sounds. However, cochlear implants have also been known to induce symptoms of tinnitus. For more information about cochlear implants, see Chapter 8.

Drug therapy

If tinnitus makes you anxious or depressed, you may want to consult your doctor about antidepressant or anti-anxiety medication. Although these types of drugs may not affect the tinnitus, they may change your perceptions of the condition and help you cope better.

In 1998 two researchers noted that about 60 percent of their tinnitus patients had major depression. The researchers conducted a study on the effects of nortriptyline (Aventyl, Pamelor), a tricyclic antidepressant, on people with tinnitus and found that it helped them sleep better, function at a higher level and feel better in general. The drug's side effects are rarely serious but may include dizziness, confusion, blurred vision, dry mouth, constipation and difficulty urinating. Older adults may experience more side effects.

Anti-anxiety medications also have been studied in people with tinnitus. Most of these drugs belong to the family of benzodiazepines, including alprazolam (Xanax), clonazepam (Klonopin) and flurazepam (Dalmane). In a 1993 study of alprazolam, participants said the tinnitus seemed less bothersome while taking the drug. The problem with alprazolam, as with other benzodiazepines, is that it can be addictive with long-term use. The drug is generally recommended for a period of no more than four months. After this period it may be helpful to use nonmedical strategies to alleviate tinnitus symptoms.

Cognitive therapy

The term *cognition* comes from the Latin word *cognoscere*, which means "to know." Cognitive therapy is a treatment approach that aims to change your understanding and perception of tinnitus rather than change the physical effects of tinnitus on you. This approach is based on the idea that negative thought patterns (cognitive distortions) can lead to negative and painful behaviors — not unlike the cycle of discomfort and frustration mentioned before.

For example, you may be convinced that your tinnitus is a sure sign of fatal disease when, in fact, tinnitus rarely indicates a serious disease, and your doctor has ruled out any such possibility. A counselor trained in cognitive therapy can help you identify and examine these disturbing notions and help you retrain your thoughts to produce a more positive and logical outlook.

Numerous studies have documented the usefulness of cognitive therapy for people with tinnitus. On many occasions this approach is used in combination with other treatments, such as drug therapy or using hearing aids.

Biofeedback

Biofeedback is a relaxation technique used to reduce the stress and anxiety so often associated with tinnitus. Like cognitive therapy, it aims to modify your response to tinnitus rather than alter the condition itself. Essentially, the method teaches you how to control bodily responses to stress. You can get biofeedback treatment in various settings, including medical centers and hospitals.

During a biofeedback session, a therapist applies electrodes and other sensors to various parts of your body. The electrodes are attached to devices that monitor your responses and give you visual or auditory feedback. For example, you might see patterns that display your blood pressure or skin temperature.

With this feedback you can learn how to produce positive changes in body functions, such as lowering your blood pressure or raising your skin temperature. These are signs of relaxation. The biofeedback therapist may use relaxation techniques to further calm you, reducing muscle tension or slowing your heart rate.

Biofeedback isn't for everyone who has tinnitus. Although it doesn't always reduce the perceived intensity of tinnitus, it may help you relax to the point where the noise is less bothersome. If you experience no improvement after a certain number of sessions, a different approach may be necessary.

Self-help tips for tinnitus

Here are measures you may consider using to reduce the severity of tinnitus and better cope with its symptoms:

Protect your hearing. Avoid loud noises, which may decrease your hearing and worsen your tinnitus. If you work in a noisy environment, wear hearing protective devices regularly.

Cover up the noise. If you're in a quiet setting where tinnitus may seem more obvious, use a masker, fan, soft music, low-volume radio or commercially available sound generator to produce soft background noise to mask the tinnitus. An FM radio set between stations generates white noise. Don't use sounds that are too loud, as they may make your tinnitus seem worse and cause additional damage to your ear.

Distract yourself. Many people say they don't hear their tinnitus if they're not paying attention to it. Do things that you enjoy and that absorb your attention. This will help take your mind off the tinnitus and provide needed relief.

Manage your stress. Stress can make your tinnitus seem worse. The basic principles of a healthy lifestyle go a long way toward reducing stress — get enough sleep and exercise, and eat a healthy diet. For example, reducing tobacco, alcohol, caffeine and salt intake may help decrease your tinnitus.

Tinnitus retraining therapy

Tinnitus retraining therapy (TRT) stems from the idea that a person can gradually lose the awareness of a sound if that sound poses no threat or demands little attention. People can become oblivious to the sound of a ticking clock or whirring fan, even a passing train. But if a sound carries some sort of meaning — for example, you associate the ticking clock with being late or behind schedule — it's likely the one you'll be most conscious of.

If you have tinnitus, you may feel a constant urge to examine and explain the sounds you're hearing and it's possible you'll never lose awareness of them. Being unable to identify the source of tinnitus may leave you feeling frustrated and insecure, which further focuses your attention on your condition.

The goal of TRT is to habituate you to your tinnitus so that the sound becomes just like other nonthreatening sounds and blends into the background. If the effort is successful, you'll perceive it less often on a conscious level.

To start treatment you use a noise generator, usually worn in your ear, for approximately eight hours a day. The device is set to a level that's audible but doesn't mask your tinnitus. You want the generator to blend the tinnitus with environmental sounds.

You'll also receive counseling that helps you perceive the condition in a rational, intelligent way so that it no longer causes fear or obsession. The audiologist will explain what's known about the tinnitus and how you can become habituated to the sound.

The therapy takes some time. Most people participate in the program for one to two years before stopping the use of the noise generator. Although it's not for everyone, about 80 percent of people who participated in a TRT program at the University of Maryland reported a decrease in the annoyance of tinnitus and in the amount of time they were aware of it.

Complementary and alternative treatments

Although Western science has yet to document all of the benefits and risks of many forms of alternative medicine, some people with tinnitus have reported relief with the use of vitamin or mineral therapy, herbal medicines and various dietary controls. Other treatments that deal with the overall well-being of your body may be helpful, such as acupuncture, acupressure, yoga, hypnosis, and joint and muscle manipulation. These usually aim to reduce the general stress of life and may help reduce anxiety.

Check with your doctor before beginning any alternative treatment. Together you can determine whether it would interact negatively with any medicines you're currently taking or affect other conditions you may have.

Part 2

The management of hearing loss

Chapter 6

Living with hearing impairment

Hearing loss isn't a physical condition that you simply can ignore, going about your daily life as if it weren't there. Hearing loss can affect every aspect of your family, work and social interactions. It can affect your self-confidence and sense of identity. For many people hearing loss is an ongoing challenge, one that can result in feeling isolated from family and friends.

It need not be this way. Your life doesn't necessarily have to change for the worse. Acknowledging your impairment as a fact of life is the first step toward overcoming and reducing the consequences of hearing loss.

Dealing with the challenges of hearing loss may also require changing some attitudes and behaviors. Many people are uncomfortable with change and find it difficult to actually make changes in life. But learning to live with your hearing loss enables you to stay engaged with your family and friends and participate in and enjoy a wide range of activities.

This chapter presents strategies for improving your ability to communicate and for finding emotional and financial support. The coping strategies described here include practical techniques such as assertive communication, speech reading and sign language. In addition, this chapter can direct you to support groups and sources of aid from community resources.

Hearing loss and quality of life

Sounds help to anchor you to the world. Sounds can give you plea-sure and contribute to a sense of belonging. Sounds can also alert you to danger or opportunity. Hearing impairment can deprive you of hearing the laughter and easy conversation between friends and family or the inspiring sounds of nature on a forest trail. Activities such as talking on the phone, eating at a restaurant, traveling, attending religious services, classes or concerts, and watching movies become more difficult for many people with hearing loss. Even something as basic as grocery shopping or running errands can pose challenges.

Hearing loss often happens gradually over several years. For that reason it may take a long time to recognize that you're having trouble hearing. Family and friends may notice your hearing loss before you do. Initially you may deny or try to minimize your impairment, perhaps because you still hear certain sounds well, or you convince yourself that other people need to speak more clearly. But denying your hearing difficulties or blaming them on external factors won't make the problem go away.

Access

Have you ever strained to understand what's being said over the public address system in an airport? Have you found yourself unable to enjoy the theater when you've been seated in a back row? Have you struggled with course work because classes are held in a lecture hall that either mutes or echoes the speaker's voice? An active life can be stressful for anyone, but it presents unique chal-lenges for people with hearing impairment.

All too often, people with hearing impairment aren't provided with the communication tools they need for travel, entertainment, education and medical care. Few movie theaters provide captioning services or other communication aids. Many clinics and hospitals don't have interpreters on staff for the hearing impaired.

Organizations such as Self Help for Hard of Hearing People (SHHH) are working to improve access in a variety of situations for people who are hearing impaired. Ongoing improvements in hear-

Denying the problem

Why do many people deny having any hearing loss and put off getting help — for years? Denial happens for many reasons:

- Hearing loss develops gradually, so you may not recognize the problem at first. You may find ways to compensate without even being aware that's what you're doing. For example, you may become more adept at lip reading.
- Many people underestimate the severity of their hearing loss. When people lose their hearing, they tend to lose the ability to hear high tones first, such as the sounds of consonants. Consonants are the sounds of speech that provide clarity and crispness. Voices may still sound loud, but they also seem mumbled.
- People often associate hearing loss and hearing aids with old age. You may fear the stigma of wearing a hearing aid.
- You may fear being considered incompetent. A common concern expressed by people coming to terms with hearing loss is that others will assume they're also losing their ability to think and act efficiently.

When you're in denial about hearing loss, you may be unable to admit to yourself that there's a problem. You may pretend that you heard what was said or that you just weren't paying attention. You may deflect attention from your hearing loss with expressions such as "You're mumbling again" or "People don't speak clearly these days" or "I don't need to hear what they're saying" or "I'm too young to need hearing aids."

Whatever the cause, denial won't help you for the long term. If you can't admit to hearing loss, you'll have trouble taking the steps to make communication easier. You'll prolong the time it takes for making adjustments and finding solutions.

ing-related assistive technology are allowing more hearing-impaired people to participate in a greater range of activities. The advent of online learning has improved access to education. For more information about assistive listening devices, captioning and other communication aids, see Chapter 9.

Employment and career

Hearing impairment may cause workplace problems. You may misunderstand an important conversation with your manager because of background noise in the office or shop. You may have difficulty comprehending someone speaking to you through a glass partition, such as at a teller's window. You may have trouble participating in meetings or conferences where several people are talking at once.

Practical solutions to many common workplace problems such as these are available. It's also useful to know your legal rights. Almost every state has a statute making it illegal to discriminate in employment on the basis of disability, race, religion, sex, age or other minority status.

Under the Americans with Disabilities Act (ADA), it's against the law to discriminate against qualified people with physical and mental disabilities in job application procedures, hiring, firing, advancement, compensation and training. The law also requires that employers make what's called reasonable accommodation for employees with disabilities. A reasonable accommodation can be any modification or adjustment to a job or work environment that will enable the employee with a disability such as hearing loss to perform essential job functions.

For deaf or severely hearing-impaired employees, reasonable accommodations may include providing a telecommunications device for the deaf (TDD), an amplified telephone or a flashing ringer on the telephone. Sound barriers or muffling can be added to control background noise in the work environment. Assistive listening systems can be installed in auditoriums and meeting rooms. The services of a transcriber or sign language interpreter can be used. In addition, employers should change or add lighting to enhance visibility.

State governments operate vocational rehabilitation agencies to help people with disabilities retain their present jobs or, if that's not possible, retrain for others. Rehabilitation means preparing someone for useful employment and successful integration into society. Certified rehabilitation counselors and rehabilitation psychologists are trained to address the work-related concerns of individuals with disabilities.

Dealing with hearing loss in the workplace

You'll benefit from the adjustments your employer makes to create a more accessible work environment, but you too can take steps to minimize problems in the workplace:

- Use the communication aids that are provided. These may include assistive listening devices such as telephone amplifiers and FM systems, captioning and alerting devices. These resources are discussed in Chapter 9.
- Move away from a source of noise. If possible, keep your desk away from busy hallways and noisy office appliances, such as air conditioners and photocopy machines.
- Ask co-workers to call you by name as they speak. This will allow you to focus your attention, understand what's being said and participate in the discussion.
- Sit upfront at meetings and presentations. Arrive early or ask to be seated close to the speaker.
- Give yourself a break in between situations that require a lot of communication. Try not to schedule meetings one after the other. Otherwise fatigue may set in.
- Alert co-workers to situations that may cause problems for you. Let them know how they can help you communicate.

Relationships and social life

Humans are social creatures — most thrive on their connections to other people. Surviving in an intensely social world can be difficult if your ability to communicate with others is hampered. Having a hearing impairment can strain your relationships with family, friends, co-workers and anyone with whom you interact daily.

For example, when you're unable to hear much of what's being said at a dinner party, you may tire quickly from the effort. This may even cause you to skip these events and stay home more often. At the store you may have trouble hearing a soft-spoken clerk. At home, when your spouse calls to you while working in front of a running faucet or dishwasher, you may not understand his or her words. Factors associated with hearing loss, such as social isolation and low self-esteem, may further strain these relationships.

Isolation. When you struggle to hear, conversations can become frustrating and tiresome. It's easy to feel isolated. Although you want to spend time with family and friends, interaction is too stressful. It's natural to avoid situations that you know will be difficult. In so doing, you cut yourself off from the world around you and the people who love you.

Social isolation is a serious problem for older adults with hearing impairment. Research by the National Council on Aging found that hearing-impaired older adults who don't use hearing aids are likely to withdraw socially, become depressed and feel that other people are getting angry with them for no reason. By contrast, hearing-impaired older adults who use hearing aids tend to have better relationships with their families and better feelings about themselves. They're more socially active, experience more interpersonal warmth, and have fewer communication difficulties and greater emotional stability.

To minimize the negative effects of hearing loss, it's important to remain socially active and involved. Casual conversations with friends or attendance at family gatherings, dinner parties, card games, and nights at the movies or theater — these are the pleasurable activities that keep us involved in the mainstream of life. Strategies to improve communication and social interaction are discussed starting on page 92.

Identity. Hearing loss can affect how you perceive your place in the world. Many adults whose hearing loss occurred early in life have, over time, incorporated the impairment into their self-images. They perceive themselves only in this way. As a result they may be accustomed to managing hearing loss in their daily lives and have developed ways to cope with it.

For adults who become hard of hearing late in life, the loss can be more disturbing and disruptive. Commonly, feelings of inadequacy accompany hearing loss and inhibit the performance of daily activities. Older adults may consider a hearing impairment as a social stigma and fear that others will treat them as incompetent. To build a new identity as an older adult with hearing loss, you may need to let go of some former attitudes about aging and appreciate the positive attributes in your life.

Psychological effects

Everyone's experience of hearing loss is different. Most people who endure any kind of serious loss, whether it's physical or emotional, go through the stages of denial, anger, bargaining, depression and acceptance. Other feelings include frustration, embarrassment and sadness. Two common psychological effects of hearing impairment are depression and anxiety.

Depression. A natural reaction to serious loss is depression. Individuals who are depressed often deny or minimize the problem. Signs and symptoms vary and don't always follow a particular pattern. But they can include persistent sadness and feelings of hopelessness, loss of appetite, sleep disturbance, extreme mood changes, irritability and poor concentration.

Many studies show a link between hearing impairment and depression. Compared with peers who have normal hearing, older adults with hearing loss report significantly more signs and symptoms of depression.

Most people with depression improve when they receive appropriate treatment with medication, counseling or both. It should be noted that depression often precedes acceptance in the stages of grief. In other words it may represent a healthy start in coming to terms with hearing loss.

Anxiety. Anxiety involves an extreme sense of fear about what may happen in the future. It often stems from misinformation and fear of the unknown. Anxiety can be influenced by other factors, such as family history, personality and general outlook on life. Anxiety and depression often go hand in hand.

Hearing impairment sets the stage for many anxiety-producing situations: On the way to a store, you may become anxious about your ability to understand the cashier. When meeting a friend, you may fear that you have misunderstood the conversation. On your own you may become anxious about your ability to hear sounds that warn you of impending threats, such as the footsteps of someone approaching around a blind corner.

Research shows that as hearing loss progresses to a moderate level, anxiety increases as well. People with hearing impairment may develop deep anxieties toward social situations in which they anticipate it will be difficult or impossible to hear others clearly. They tend to avoid these situations at all costs.

If you're concerned that you or someone you care about may have an anxiety disorder, talk to your doctor or a mental health professional. Treatment can help manage the anxiety.

Strategies for social interaction

Although hearing loss may affect your relationships, many strategies and tools are available to help you communicate effectively and stay involved in a range of activities.

As you're learning new communication skills, you may work with health care professionals, other people with hearing loss, family and friends. Most people are willing and able to help you communicate better, and it's wise to accept their assistance. But you can be more than a passive recipient of services. Take control of your own listening needs. It requires commitment and effort to learn as much as you can about effective communication.

Your communication can improve over time even if you don't hear each and every sound or word. Your remaining hearing, along with visual information, context clues and life experience, can help you to understand speech and to communicate. With the assistance of modern technology, the impact of hearing loss on your life can be considerably reduced.

Assertive communication
Good communication may require that you become more assertive. That doesn't mean becoming loud and bossy. Assertiveness simply means speaking out for and working toward meeting your needs without ignoring other people's needs in the process. Often with hearing loss, you'll need to practice assertiveness in order to ensure effective communication.

Assertive communication means directly expressing how you feel and what you need. With assertive communication, you:
- Let others know that you have a hearing loss. Then they won't misconstrue your behavior or think you're aloof or forgetful.

- Are aware that your hearing loss affects other people and are prepared to deal with their reactions.
- Use hearing aids and assistive listening devices.
- Ask for, but not demand, help when you need it.
- Tell people exactly what you need. For example, you might say "Sorry, I don't hear as well as I used to. Would you mind speaking a little louder?" You might ask someone to slow his or her speech, look at you, move a hand from the face, or repeat a phrase.
- Postpone conversation when you're tired.
- Give feedback to show your appreciation.
- Are willing to admit if you're taking out your emotions on someone else.
- Modify your environment to fit your hearing needs.

By making the effort to communicate assertively, you'll probably find it easier to deal with many social situations. Most people are receptive if you tell them you're having trouble hearing and will ask what they can do to help.

An environment conducive to better hearing
One of the most effective strategies for improving communication and social interaction is to avoid or modify situations that make hearing difficult. Often, by altering or stage-managing your environment, you can avoid communication breakdowns. You can achieve this in several ways:

Move closer to a source of sound you want to hear. This may include a television or stereo, a speaker at a meeting or worship service, or guests in your home. Arrange furniture so that guests or family members are nearby and facing directly toward you. In locations where you can't rearrange the furniture, choose your seating for minimum distance and maximum visibility.

Move away from distracting or overpowering noise. Try to avoid seating in locations close to machinery and appliances or busy passageways. In a restaurant, request a booth or table away from the kitchen, lobby, bar or other noisy spot. Try to avoid sitting close to music speakers or ventilation ducts. At home turn off the television or radio when you're conversing with someone.

Position yourself so that the speaker's face is visible and well lit. Visual clues, such as facial expression or position of the head, can provide a clear context for what's being said.

Plan in advance for social activities. Before you attend an event in a busy or crowded area, such as a theater or place of worship, call ahead to see if the facility has assistive listening devices available. Arrive early so that you have a choice of seats.

Speech reading

Speech reading, also called lip reading, is a tool that someone with hearing impairment can use to navigate social situations. Speech reading is a technique for recognizing spoken words by watching the movements of a speaker's lips, tongue, lower jaw, eyes and eyebrows, as well as facial expressions, body stances and gestures. These provide important visual clues to the spoken message.

Many people, whether they hear normally or not, rely on speech reading to some degree. In fact, most of them are unaware that they're speech reading. For example, when background noise is loud, people with normal hearing instinctively try to match the motion of the speaker's lips to the sounds they can hear. For people who have a hearing loss, including those who use hearing aids, speech sounds are quieter, distorted or both. Speech reading allows them to follow conversation more easily. Some people who are profoundly deaf choose to communicate using speech reading and speech rather than sign language.

Speech reading works best if you have some hearing left and use a hearing aid or other assistive listening device. It's accomplished primarily by following lip patterns — the shapes made by people's mouths when they speak. For example, the vowel *o* is formed with rounded lips, and the consonant *m* is made by pressing the lips firmly together. Even the most skilled speech reader can't pick up every word. Not all sounds are visible on the lips, and some sounds look exactly alike. For example, *b*, *m* and *p* look similar on the lips. So the words *ban*, *man* and *pan* are almost impossible to distinguish.

Many other factors — fast speech, poor pronunciation, bad lighting, an averted face, a covered mouth, a moustache and beard — can make speech reading difficult or impossible. Therefore, you often need to rely on the context of the sentence and other nonverbal cues to understand what's being said.

Speech reading skills usually improve with practice. The more you learn, the more confident you'll become with your ability to communicate. Although it's not the whole answer for dealing with hearing impairment, many people become proficient speech readers and find that it keeps the door open to social interaction.

Learning speech reading. You can learn speech reading in several ways. Try different methods until you find one that works for you. As with learning any new skill, learning to identify the basic sounds for speech reading takes time and patience.

Methods to learn speech reading include:

Self-practice with a handbook. Watch yourself speak in front of a mirror, progressing at your own pace.

Practice with a friend or family member. This may involve informal conversation or specific training exercises.

Use videotapes or audiotapes. These materials have the advantage of easy replay. Repetition is crucial for learning.

Attend speech reading classes. Many people benefit from learning in a supportive atmosphere from a qualified teacher. This can keep you motivated and give you a chance to talk with other people who have a hearing loss.

Tips for speech reading. The goal of speech reading is better communication. Rather than trying to catch every word that's spoken, focus on the overall intent and context. Here are suggestions for making speech reading easier:

- Position yourself so that a light source is behind you and the speaker's face is clearly visible. Any factor that reduces the visibility of the lips will interfere with speech reading.
- Identify the topic being discussed as quickly as possible. If you're familiar with the topic and can identify key words, you won't need to analyze every phrase.
- Watch for clues in the speaker's facial expressions, body language and gestures.
- Before you enter a conversation, inform the person who's speaking that you have hearing loss. Ask the person not to shout, exaggerate mouth movements, chew gum or talk fast.

- Try to relax as much as possible. Don't try to understand everything, or you may become tense, which can make speech reading more difficult.
- Use your remaining hearing in combination with speech reading. Diminish background noise by turning off the television or radio, closing the door or window, or sitting in a quiet section of a restaurant.
- Focus on the message rather than specific lip movements. You'll find that subsequent sentences may clarify the words and sentences you've missed.
- If you can't fill in a missing word, ask the speaker to rephrase the sentence.
- Take frequent breaks, especially when you're first learning to speech read. The technique requires deep concentration, and you may tire quickly. When you get the chance, close your eyes and relax for a few minutes.

Communicating with a hearing-impaired person

Communication is the lifeblood of any relationship. When you're conversing with someone who's hearing impaired, keep in mind that what to you is simple communication may be a tiring effort for your companion. He or she has to make an active effort to understand. A hearing aid may help, but turning up the volume won't make distorted sounds any clearer.

You can enhance communication with a hearing-impaired person by following a few practical suggestions:

- Before starting to talk, reduce the level of background noise. Turn off the television, radio, air conditioner or other noisy appliances. Don't leave a faucet running. If you can't reduce background noise, try to move to a quieter area.
- Make sure you have the person's attention before speaking. You can do this by saying his or her name or touching his or her shoulder.
- Talk face to face. Speak at eye level, and no more than a few feet away. Don't chew gum, smoke, talk behind a newspaper or cover your mouth while you're speaking.

Sign language

Many deaf people communicate using sign language. Sign language uses hand signs — made with hand shape, position and movement — as well as body movements, gestures, facial expressions and other visual cues to form words.

Different sign languages are used in different countries or regions. American Sign Language (ASL) is commonly used in the United States and Canada. It's a complete, complex language with its own grammatical rules and semantics. Like English, ASL allows for regional differences and jargon.

Facial expressions and body movements are very important in sign language. For example, English speakers usually signal a question by using a particular tone of voice, but ASL users do so by raising the eyebrows and widening the eyes.

Learning sign language. Learning sign language takes time. Picking up enough signs for basic communication can take a year

- Speak at a normal conversational level, especially if the person is wearing a hearing aid or has a cochlear implant. Don't shout. If necessary, modestly increase your volume.
- Speak clearly but naturally. Slow your speech a little, using a few more pauses than usual.
- Use facial expressions, gestures and other body language to make your points.
- Watch your listener's face for signs that comprehension is a problem. Rephrase your statements if the listener is unsure of what's been said.
- Alert your listener to changes in topics of conversation.
- Show extra consideration in a group situation. What's known as cross talk is one of the most difficult situations for someone with hearing loss. Try to structure the event so that only one person is speaking at a time. At meetings it's helpful to display an agenda on a board or overhead transparency and, as the meeting progresses, to indicate which item is under discussion.

or more. Community colleges, universities, libraries, churches, and organizations for deaf and hard of hearing people offer sign language classes. Qualified ASL teachers are certified by a national professional organization, the American Sign Language Teachers Association (ASLTA). The ASLTA Web site (*www.aslta.org*) has information about state and local chapters.

Hearing dogs

You're probably familiar with guide dogs for people who are blind. Did you know that service dogs are also available to help those who have severe or profound hearing loss? Hearing dogs are trained to alert individuals to such sounds as a knock at the door, a ringing telephone, an oven timer, an alarm clock, a car horn, and smoke and fire alarms.

Hearing dogs don't bark to get your attention. Rather, they're trained to use their nose or paw to nudge you, then lead you to the source of the sound. Hearing dogs can also carry messages or notes between you and another household member. They can warn of a vehicle approaching from behind or making a sudden turn.

According to the Americans with Disabilities Act, hearing dogs must be allowed to accompany their owners into businesses and other places that serve the public. Often a bright orange or yellow leash identifies a hearing dog. But the dog doesn't have to have special identification to accompany you into a business.

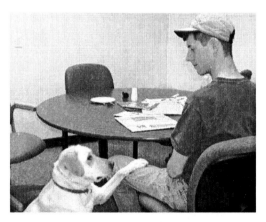 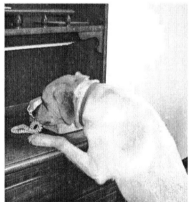

To alert you to a sound, a hearing dog will first nudge you to get your attention (left), then lead you to the source of the sound, such as a ringing telephone (right).

Getting a hearing dog. Hearing dogs come in all shapes and sizes. Many are taken from animal shelters and given three to six months of training. There's no national standard for training the dogs, and they're not required to be certified. Some people with a hearing impairment choose to work directly with a private trainer and the dog, and others prefer to get a dog that's already trained. But you may have to wait two or more years to get one.

In the United States the two largest hearing dog agencies are Paws With A Cause (PAWS) and Canine Companions for Independence (CCI). Most service-dog organizations are nonprofits that provide the dogs at no charge to the people who need them.

Finding support

Even under the best circumstances, living with a hearing impairment will have frustrating moments. There will be times when you feel overwhelmed by the effort of staying connected to the hearing world or isolated by your inability to hear certain sounds. You don't have to cope with all of the challenges alone. Various options to receive support are available for people with hearing loss, such as aural rehabilitation or a support group. Many national, state and local organizations provide practical information on hearing and resources for living with hearing impairment.

Aural rehabilitation

If you don't feel comfortable with your hearing impairment, consider aural rehabilitation, also called hearing rehabilitation. Aural rehabilitation focuses on your adjustment to hearing loss and tries to reduce the difficulties. Its advocates say that by making the best use of hearing aids and assistive listening devices, you can begin to take charge of your communication needs.

An audiologist, a speech-language pathologist or both typically provide these services. You may work one-on-one with a therapist, as part of a group or in both settings. Participating in group therapy can be especially helpful because you'll meet others facing the same issues as you are.

The overall goal of aural rehabilitation is to maximize your self-confidence and your ability to communicate in everyday situations. This may be achieved by:

• Understanding your hearing loss
• Learning how to listen
• Learning skills in speech reading
• Building confidence in communication situations
• Dealing with emotional problems related to hearing loss
• Learning about different types of hearing aids and assistive listening devices
• Understanding legal rights and being your own advocate
• Promoting your family's understanding of your needs
• Making it easier for your family to communicate with you

A typical rehabilitation session lasts from one to two hours a week. The session may be held at a medical clinic, rehabilitation center, community college or private office. Aural rehabilitation sessions generally last over a period of four to 10 weeks.

Support groups

Getting together with people who are experiencing the same things you are is a good way to find support. Belonging to a group can remind you that you're not the only one with hearing loss. Participating in a support group gives you the opportunity to learn and share knowledge. Support groups aren't the same as group aural rehabilitation. An audiologist leads an aural rehabilitation group. Peers frequently lead support groups.

Support groups are an excellent resource for problem solving and mutual support. They're also a way to meet potential new friends. How have others handled traveling, meetings, telephone conversations, communicating in public places or dealing with difficult work colleagues? What problems have they had with hearing aids? Have they used assistive listening devices?

Many national organizations with local chapters provide support groups for people with hearing loss. These include the Alexander Graham Bell Association for the Deaf and Hard of Hearing, the Association of Late-Deafened Adults, the Cochlear Implant Association, the National Association of the Deaf, and a

---

Evaluating information

You can find hundreds of products, publications, services and Web sites devoted to hearing impairment. But be careful. The information ranges from solid research to outright quackery.

When evaluating information you find on the Internet, consider these guidelines:

- Look for Web sites created by national organizations, universities, government agencies or major medical centers.
- Look for current information. Search for the most recent information you can find.
- Check for the information source. Notice whether articles refer to published research. Look for a board of qualified professionals who review the content before it's published. Be wary of commercial sites or personal testimonials that push a single point of view.
- Double-check the information. Visit several sites and compare the information offered.

---

group called Self Help for Hard of Hearing People (SHHH). See "Additional resources" at the back of this book for contact information for these organizations.

National, state and local resources

Dozens of national, state and local organizations provide services for people who are deaf or hard of hearing. These resources include advocacy, education, financial aid, information and referral, advice on medical issues, and counseling on professional and work issues. There are also opportunities for self-help and support groups, recreational and social activities, and spiritual needs. Most organizations have Web sites and publications about hearing loss that offer clear, easy-to-understand information for the general public.

The federal government provides information on affirmative action programs, reasonable accommodation and means to improve accessibility for disabled persons. For example, if you feel your legal rights have been violated, you may contact the Equal Employment Opportunity Commission for advice.

States provide services for individuals who are deaf and hard of hearing. The state office might be a commission or a vocational rehabilitation program for people with disabilities. Offices that provide rehabilitation services often provide counseling and job retraining and may help pay for hearing aids. Some states have programs to provide amplified telephones to people with a hearing impairment. A state human rights or human relations commission or a governor's committee on employment of people with disabilities can provide information on related laws.

Chapter 7

Hearing aids

Hearing loss need not mean you're cut off from the world of sound. If you feel like you're missing out and want to hear better, you'll likely benefit from using a hearing aid. Hearing aids can't restore normal hearing, but they can definitely improve your ability to communicate and respond to sound. These tiny, sophisticated electronic devices are the single-most effective treatment for the majority of people with hearing loss.

Hearing aids can greatly enhance your ability to interact with others. They can minimize many problems that go along with hearing loss, such as difficulty understanding conversations or hearing timers and beepers. And they can help combat feelings of social isolation and problems with self-image.

Hearing aid technology has improved tremendously in the last two decades. Years ago hearing aids were large and cumbersome. They had a harsh, distorted sound quality, like a cheap transistor radio. Newer hearing aids are compact and provide far better sound quality. An array of choices is available to match your lifestyle with your communication needs.

Over time you'll adjust to your hearing aid and enjoy your enhanced ability to hear and communicate in a variety of situations. By wearing your hearing aid regularly and taking good care of it, you'll likely notice improvements in your quality of life.

Setting priorities and realistic expectations

Motivation is the key to success with hearing aids. People who have a positive attitude and want to hear better are often better hearing aid users. They're also more likely to continue wearing them. If you decide to get a hearing aid, selecting which type to use is an individual process based on your specific needs. Each person and each type of hearing loss is quite different. In making your selection, it helps to be informed, patient and open to the suggestions of your hearing aid dispenser.

You can do several things to increase your satisfaction with hearing aids. You've probably already taken the first steps — acknowledging your hearing loss and being willing to seek a solution to the challenges it presents.

It's also important to establish your priorities about what you want from a hearing aid. Identify situations in which communication is most difficult for you. When is it important for you to hear especially well? Are there times when you concentrate so hard to hear that you become fatigued? Your priority may be to hear your children or grandchildren when they come to visit, or to understand conversation during your weekly card game.

When you buy a hearing aid, you'll typically face trade-offs among many factors, such as performance, style, size, technology and cost. You may want the smallest device that works for you. Maybe you want a hearing aid that's easy to handle and operate. If you spend most of your time at home by yourself, you may not need the latest, most expensive brand. Prepare a list of your priorities, ranking various considerations by order of importance.

Another key to satisfaction is keeping your expectations realistic. Everyone experiences varying degrees of success with hearing aids. If you expect a hearing aid to give you perfect hearing, you'll be disappointed. How well a hearing aid functions for you will depend on several variables, including the severity of your hearing loss, the situations in which you want to hear better and your motivation.

One way to develop realistic expectations is to educate yourself about hearing loss. Another is to talk to others with hearing loss. It's also important to work closely with a hearing aid dispenser.

Why do people resist wearing hearing aids?
Despite the benefits of hearing aids, many people with hearing loss haven't even tried them. Studies indicate that only about one in five of the estimated 30 million Americans with hearing loss uses a hearing aid. People reject the idea of wearing aids for many reasons, including an unwillingness to accept hearing loss, the cost of the devices and reports of bad experiences with hearing aids from friends or relatives. Often the biggest deterrent is fear of the social stigma — concern that a hearing aid will be considered a sign of old age, incompetence, inferiority or unattractiveness.

Such concerns have little basis in fact. Studies have investigated whether hearing aids actually make people look older. Research found that, indeed, hearing aids might make adults look older — but by less than one year, a difference so small as to have no practical significance.

In addition, the advances in technology and design are making hearing aids stylistically more appealing and functionally more effective. As technology has advanced, so has users' satisfaction with hearing aids.

Getting a hearing aid may require an attitude change. You'll need to weigh the benefits of wearing a hearing aid against the obstacles of being unable to hear people speaking. You'll need to accept that a hearing aid isn't a sign of aging and dependence. It'll enhance your communication with others and help you stay connected and involved.

What hearing aids can and can't do

Hearing aids can improve your hearing. They do so by making sounds louder and allowing more sounds to be heard. You should be able to understand spoken words with less strain. It should be easier to hear people talking in a soft voice. You'll probably be able to turn the television sound down to a level that's more comfortable for others in the room who don't have hearing loss. Hearing aids can also help you hear more environmental sounds, which gives you a better sense of your surroundings.

Hearing aids can allow you to hear in some situations in which you previously had difficulty hearing, such as attending the theater or services at a worship hall. They can help you feel more at ease when you're on your own — for example, while shopping — or in situations where speakers may not talk directly to you.

Although hearing aids can improve your hearing, they won't restore a completely natural sound. They're electronic devices that can slightly change the quality of what you hear, just as a radio does. When you first listen through a hearing aid, you'll notice that many things sound a little different. You'll likely adapt to this quickly. Furthermore, hearing loss causes the ear to distort some of the sounds you hear. Hearing aids can't eliminate that distortion, so those sounds may not be crystal clear.

You may still have problems understanding speech in certain situations. When there's a lot of background noise or many people talking at once, hearing aids can't separate a voice that you want to hear from other voices or sounds you don't want to hear. Remember that even with normal hearing, background noise can interfere with your understanding of speech.

Newer hearing aids have features that attempt to help in noisy situations. These attachments are discussed on page 114. As hearing aid technology continues to improve, more efforts will be made to help with difficult listening situations.

How a hearing aid works

Many types of hearing aids are available, and the technology is continually improving. But the fundamental purpose of all hearing aids is the same: to make sounds louder.

All hearing aids work by collecting sounds from the environment via a small microphone, amplifying the sounds and then directing this amplified signal into the user's ear via a loudspeaker. The amplified signal stimulates the inner ear, which activates nerve fibers that carry the sound impulses to your brain.

The illustration on page 107 labels the parts of what's known as an in-the-ear style of hearing aid.

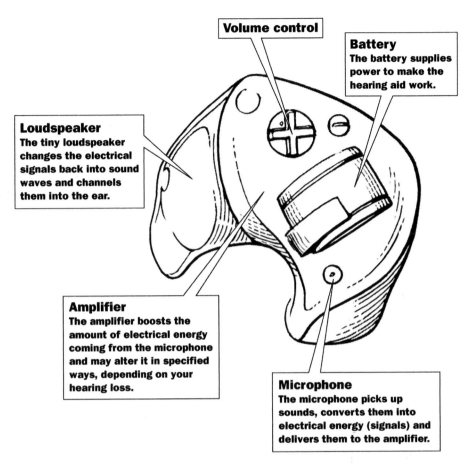

Volume control

Battery
The battery supplies power to make the hearing aid work.

Loudspeaker
The tiny loudspeaker changes the electrical signals back into sound waves and channels them into the ear.

Amplifier
The amplifier boosts the amount of electrical energy coming from the microphone and may alter it in specified ways, depending on your hearing loss.

Microphone
The microphone picks up sounds, converts them into electrical energy (signals) and delivers them to the amplifier.

The components of this in-the-ear style of hearing aid are held in a small plastic container called the casing. In a behind-the-ear style of hearing aid, the casing rests behind the ear and is connected to an earmold (earpiece) by a plastic tube. The earmold is custom-made to fit into the ear and direct sound into the ear canal.

Selecting a hearing aid

When selecting a hearing aid, your decisions involve style, size and circuitry features, as well as whether to use one or two devices. This may become confusing because the decisions can be made somewhat independently of each another. For example, you may have heard that digital hearing aids provide the best sound. What may not be clear is that *digital* refers to the technology of the electrical components and not to a particular style of hearing aid. Style and circuitry — along with size — are separate issues. Any circuitry can be placed in any style of hearing aid.

Are two hearing aids better than one?

Can you hear better with a hearing aid in each ear? The answer, in most cases, is yes. Wearing two (binaural) hearing aids has many advantages over wearing one (monaural) aid. More information is going to your brain, and the signals reaching each ear are slightly different. This can make it easier to hear speech in situations with background noise.

Two aids also provide more-balanced hearing. You won't have a bad side, where the sound is muted. Having two ears to listen with helps you to localize sound more easily, so you won't have to spin your head around to figure out who's talking. Another advantage of wearing two aids is that neither of the devices needs to be turned up as loudly as when wearing only one. This helps reduce feedback and increases comfort.

Financial constraints and inability to wear an aid in one ear keep some people from wearing two aids. Talk to your audiologist or hearing aid dealer about your options.

Hearing aid electronics

The *circuitry* of hearing aids refers to what's inside — the technology of the electronic components. Hearing aid electronics are designed or programmed to amplify certain frequencies more than others. The frequencies chosen for amplification will compensate for the corresponding damaged hair cells in the cochlea. The frequency range to which a hearing aid is programmed is called the frequency response. Hearing aid circuitry may be basic analog, programmable analog or digital.

Basic analog. These conventional hearing aids contain analog electronic components. Analog is a type of electrical signal — an electrical copy of the sound waves in the environment. The analog signal is then amplified so that it can be heard better.

An audiologist or hearing aid dealer will select different components and settings based on your hearing loss. If the hearing aid has a volume control, you can adjust it yourself. This type of circuitry is probably more appropriate for people who do most of their communicating in relatively quiet situations.

Advantages. This can be the least expensive technology.

Disadvantages. These aids are generally not as flexible as programmable analog or digital hearing aids for adjusting to a particular type of hearing loss and to specific hearing needs. Because the processing is less sophisticated, these aids may be less effective in difficult listening environments.

Programmable analog. These aids have analog circuitry, but they can be digitally programmed on a computer to permit a variety of settings for different types of hearing loss and hearing needs. The hearing aid dispenser programs the settings and later fine-tunes them to your hearing loss and changes in your hearing. Some of these hearing aids will have multiple programs. This may allow you to adjust them to your situation with a remote control or by pushing a small button on the hearing aid.

Advantages. Many programmable analog devices offer more flexibility than do basic analog aids, with more adjustments for the amplification of soft sounds without overamplifying loud sounds. Those with multiple programs allow you to adjust the response of the hearing aid to different listening situations.

Disadvantages. They can be more expensive than basic analog.

Digital. In these aids the amplifying of sound is handled by a computer chip rather than conventional analog circuitry. This type of aid converts incoming sound into digital code, then analyzes and adjusts the sound based on the user's hearing loss and listening needs. This information is stored in a computer program within the aid. Then the signals are converted back into sound waves and delivered to your ears. The result is sound that's more finely tuned to your hearing loss.

Advantages. This is the most advanced and versatile technology. Some digital aids may have added features that perform better in noisy situations than analog devices do.

Disadvantages. This is the most expensive circuitry. It may be more than you need. When you're using a cell phone, you may experience more static or interference with this type of hearing aid than you would with either of the other types. Fortunately, the manufacturers of cell phones and of hearing aids are making progress in resolving this problem.

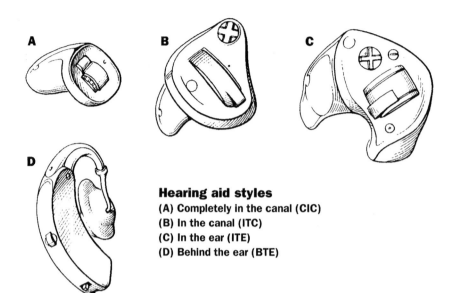

Hearing aid styles
(A) Completely in the canal (CIC)
(B) In the canal (ITC)
(C) In the ear (ITE)
(D) Behind the ear (BTE)

Hearing aid styles

Hearing aids come in various styles, which differ in size and the way they're placed in the ear. Some are small enough to fit deeply in the ear canal, making them almost invisible. The most widely sold aids are those that fit partially in the ear canal or in the bowl of the outer ear. You can get basic analog, programmable analog or digital technology in any hearing aid style.

Generally, the smaller a hearing aid is, the less powerful it is, the shorter its battery life and the more it will cost. Smaller aids may be more likely to produce feedback. Feedback refers to a high-pitched whistle and other noise that's made when amplified sound inadvertently is picked up by the microphone and re-amplified. This is similar to the noise you may hear over a public-address system if the volume is too high. New technology is helping to reduce the feedback problem in hearing aids.

With so many styles of hearing aids to choose from, keep in mind that the choice of style concerns more than just looks. The style that's right for you will depend largely on your hearing test results. Usually, the greater your hearing loss, the larger your hearing aid will need to be. And some styles of hearing aids tend to not work as well if your hearing is good for lower frequencies but decreases substantially at higher frequencies.

The size and shape of your ear and ear canal may eliminate other style options. The in-the-canal styles can be difficult to fit on smaller ears. Your ability to handle a small hearing aid style may be a factor, especially if you have limited finger dexterity. Medical conditions also may dictate which style is appropriate.

Completely in the canal. The smallest hearing aid available is called a completely-in-the-canal (CIC) aid. All parts, including the battery, are contained in a tiny case that fits deep inside the ear canal. A thin, plastic pull cord sticks out into the bowl-shaped area of the ear to help in removal. The CIC aid is appropriate for mild to moderate hearing loss. It's not used for children or infants.

Advantages. This is the least visible hearing aid. It may help reduce wind noise.

Disadvantages. This is the least powerful hearing aid style and isn't appropriate for more severe hearing loss. CIC aids have less space for add-ons such as volume control or directional microphones. In addition, batteries are smaller, so battery life may be shorter. This style of hearing aid is more expensive than other styles.

In the canal. An in-the-canal (ITC) hearing aid fits partly in the ear canal but not as deeply as a CIC aid. The edge of the ITC aid extends into the bowl of the ear. ITC aids can accommodate mild to moderately severe hearing loss, but they're not appropriate for infants and children.

Advantages. Like CIC aids, ITC aids are hardly noticeable. An ITC aid is potentially more powerful than a CIC aid, with more opportunity for add-ons.

Disadvantages. ITC aids can be difficult to handle and insert and for replacing batteries. They're also rather expensive.

In the ear. An in-the-ear (ITE) style of hearing aid fills most of the bowl-shaped area of your outer ear. ITE aids are appropriate for mild to severe hearing loss.

Advantages. These aids can be more powerful than those that fit in the canal, and they can accommodate more add-ons, such as a telecoil and directional microphones. They're appropriate for a wide range of hearing loss. Their battery is slightly larger and easier to insert than that of the in-the-canal styles.

Disadvantages. ITE aids may pick up more wind noise.

Behind the ear. Behind-the-ear (BTE) aids have two parts. A small plastic case that rests behind the ear contains the hearing aid circuitry: the microphone, amplifier and loudspeaker. The case is connected by plastic tubing to a custom-made earmold (earpiece) that directs the amplified sound into your ear. BTE aids are appropriate for almost all types of hearing loss and for people of all ages.

BTE aids are often erroneously perceived as old-fashioned or not technologically advanced. But in fact, BTE aids have modern electronic and digital technology like the other styles and in some cases provide the greatest improvement in hearing.

Advantages. These are the most powerful hearing aids, and they can be adjusted for any degree of hearing loss. BTE aids are the best style for infants, children and people with more severe hearing loss. BTE aids are also the easiest to maintain, partly because battery replacement is easier. These aids usually require fewer repairs.

Disadvantages. Some people don't have enough space between their ear and the side of their head to accommodate this style. This type may pick up more wind noise than the smaller aids do.

Disposable. One of the newer options in hearing aids is disposable aids. Their sound quality can be as good as standard aids, and they offer easier maintenance. Disposable aids are in-the-canal hearing aids designed to be worn for about 40 to 70 days, then discarded and replaced with fresh devices.

Using disposable aids may eliminate maintenance problems due to moisture and wax buildup that occur with ongoing use of standard aids. Battery replacement problems also are avoided.

Disposable devices can be fitted at the hearing evaluation appointment, so you can leave wearing your new hearing aid. With standard hearing aids, a mold of your ear is made, and a second appointment is needed for fitting. However, disposable aids won't fit everyone's ears or meet everyone's hearing needs.

Advantages. Disposable aids require minimal maintenance. You can receive them at the time of your hearing evaluation.

Disadvantages. They're not custom fit to the ear and may not fit everyone comfortably. They have less adjustable circuitry and no special features. Also, there's the ongoing expense of purchasing a new aid every other month.

Implantable. Implantable hearing aids are an alternative to standard hearing aids for people with moderate to severe sensorineural hearing loss, that is, loss associated with damage to the inner ear. These devices operate differently from other hearing aids. Standard hearing aids convert sound into electrical signals and amplify them. Implantable devices work on principles of mechanical vibration. They conduct sound by vibrating the middle ear bones directly to stimulate the inner ear. The devices aren't recommended for people with conductive hearing loss — hearing loss in the outer ear or middle ear — and with active or recurrent middle ear infections.

Implantable hearing aids use a tiny electromagnet attached to the bones of the middle ear and an external unit that stimulates the magnet. Fully implantable devices are still under development. For some units a receiver is surgically implanted into the skull behind the ear. An external amplifier is held in place by a magnet over the implanted receiver. A wire leads from the receiver to the electromagnet attached to one of the middle ear bones. Other units have an external processor containing both amplifier and receiver that's worn in or behind the ear, similar to standard hearing aid styles.

Implantable aids are put in place during an outpatient surgical procedure that lasts from 30 minutes to two hours.

Advantages. These devices are expected to produce a clearer, more natural sound, although research hasn't yet confirmed this.

Disadvantages. Implantable aids require surgery, and the procedure is expensive — $6,000 to $18,000 per ear, depending on which device is selected and on which type of anesthesia is necessary.

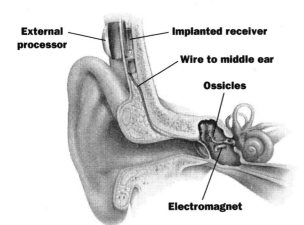

External processor

Implanted receiver

Wire to middle ear

Ossicles

Electromagnet

In some styles of implantable hearing aids, an external processor collects sound and transmits it to an implanted receiver. The receiver transmits the signal through a wire to the electromagnet, which stimulates the ossicles.

Special features

Another consideration when choosing a hearing aid is special add-on features that can help you in difficult listening situations.

Directional microphones. Most hearing aids are equipped with an omnidirectional microphone, which picks up sounds from the sides and behind as well as in front of the wearer. A directional microphone picks up and amplifies the sound directly in front of you more than it does the sounds from other directions. This can improve your understanding of private conversations in noisy environments. A hearing aid may have a microphone with two sound inlets or have multiple microphones. Either arrangement may allow you to switch between directional and omnidirectional modes. All but the CIC aid can have directional microphones.

Telecoils. Many BTE hearing aids, and some ITE and ITC aids, contain a built-in telecoil circuit that can be activated by a switch or button on the hearing aid. Telecoils relay a voice on the telephone receiver using an electromagnetic signal rather than using an acoustic signal, which can cause feedback (whistling) with some hearing aids. Telecoils also interface with a variety of assistive listening devices. (See Chapter 9 for more information on these devices.) Telecoils may not work with cell phones.

Audio-input options. An input jack on your hearing aid allows you to connect a wire directly to a television, stereo, separate microphone or assistive listening device.

Ear-level FM systems. FM listening devices are particularly helpful for overcoming the effects of noise, reverberation and distance from a speaker. Some BTE hearing aids combine the circuitry and an FM receiver within the same case. The FM receiver responds to the signal from a specially designed, hand-held FM transmitter. FM devices are discussed in more detail in Chapter 9.

Purchasing a hearing aid

Audiologists and hearing aid dealers, sometimes called hearing instrument specialists, sell hearing aids. Most states require all hearing aid dispensers to be licensed, which means that they've passed written and practical tests in the field. Audiologists have a graduate degree in audiology, are certified by either the American Speech-Language-Hearing Association or the American Academy of Audiology and are licensed by the state in which they practice. The practices of some ear, nose and throat doctors, also referred to as ENTs or otolaryngologists, include audiologists to provide testing and rehabilitation services and to dispense hearing aids.

Although hearing aid dealers aren't required to have a college degree, many complete a distance learning course, pass a state-administered exam, and are licensed or registered by the state they work in. They should be certified by the National Board for Certification in Hearing Instrument Sciences.

It's critical that you find a reputable, honest, qualified hearing aid dispenser. Start by asking your doctor or people you know for recommendations. In addition, you can get lists of hearing aid dispensers in your area by contacting professional organizations such as the American Academy of Audiology, the American Speech-Language-Hearing Association and the International Society of Hearing Instrument Specialists. Several Internet sites sell hearing aids, referring you to dispensers within their network, but this practice is illegal in a number of states. Don't buy hearing aids by mail or over the Internet from makers who claim you don't need to see a dispenser in person.

Discuss hearing aid options thoroughly with your audiologist or hearing aid dealer. Make sure you understand why a specific type of hearing aid is being recommended and how you can expect it to meet your needs.

Regardless of what style or type of hearing aid you buy, always purchase it with a return privilege. The aid should come with a 30- to 60-day adjustment period and a return policy. You may need that much time to get used to the device and decide if it helps you sufficiently to retain the aid.

Steps in buying a hearing aid
In the discussion that follows, the terms *hearing aid* and *aid* are used in the singular form. But keep in mind that most often greater improvement is achieved with a hearing aid in each ear.

Before you buy a hearing aid, plan to be examined by a physician, preferably an ear, nose and throat doctor. The Food and Drug Administration (FDA) requires dispensers to obtain proof from you that you've had a physician evaluate your hearing within the past six months before selling you a hearing aid, or to have you sign a waiver. An examination can determine whether medical treatment can improve your hearing or if a medical condition prevents you from using a hearing aid.

Also plan a complete examination of your hearing by an audiologist. Get a copy of your audiogram if you'll not be buying your hearing aid at the place where you're tested. The audiogram provides an accurate guide for selecting your hearing aid.

Discuss your needs and expectations with your hearing aid dispenser. Specify which situations cause you the greatest amount of hearing difficulty. The goal is to match your lifestyle and your communication needs as closely as possible.

After gathering information about your hearing abilities and your preferences, the dispenser will discuss various options with you and offer some recommendations. Before you make a final decision, be sure you understand the features and cost of your selection, and the terms of the trial period and return policy.

Once you've made a selection, your dispenser will fit the aid. For most types of aids, the dispenser will take an impression of your ear, using a putty-like material to create an accurate mold of its shape. This enables the manufacturer to make a hearing aid that is comfortable and fits properly. You'll return to the dispenser's office in one to two weeks for the fitting. This visit also involves programming or adjusting the aid to provide maximum help for your hearing loss.

Once the aid is fitted, the dispenser should instruct you on operating and maintaining the aid — how to insert and remove it, check the battery, adjust the controls and otherwise care for it. Be sure to ask the dispenser any questions you have.

The adjustment period allows you to get used to wearing the aid. You'll probably schedule a return visit to the dispenser within a few weeks to have your progress checked. Until that time, write down questions that occur to you and take them to your appoint-

Tips for purchasing a hearing aid

Keep these suggestions in mind when selecting a hearing aid:

- With all of the options available, more than one type of hearing aid could work for you. If one or more features of your first selection prove unsatisfactory, inquire about trying out a different type of hearing aid.
- Don't assume that the newest, most expensive model is best for you. A less expensive aid might improve your hearing just as much as other models.
- Be cautious of "free" consultations and dispensers who sell only one brand of hearing aid. Look for a dispenser who deals with several hearing aid manufacturers so that you'll have plenty of options.
- Be alert to misleading claims. Be wary of manufacturers who say their hearing aids can eliminate background noise. Some aids can make hearing in noisy places more comfortable, but no aids can filter out one voice from other voices in a crowded room.
- Ask what the cost of the aid includes. Most dispensers bundle into a single fee the cost of the hearing aid and other related costs, such as those for a certain number of follow-up visits, the warranty and one pack of batteries.
- Be sure to get the terms of the adjustment period and warranty in writing. This should include the return policy, the exact amount to be refunded if you return the aid, how long the warranty lasts (preferably one or two years) and specifically what is and isn't covered — it should cover both parts and labor.
- During the trial period, keep a detailed list of what you like or dislike about your hearing aid. Take the list with you when you return to the dispenser.

ment so that you can have them answered. If during the 30- to 60-day period you can't adjust to the aid or you decide that you don't benefit from using it, notify your dispenser. Under the trial period agreement, you're entitled to a refund for the cost of the device.

Costs of hearing aids

The cost of hearing aids varies considerably. A good basic analog hearing aid ranges from $600 to $1,500. A programmable analog aid costs about $750 to $1,900, and a digital aid ranges from $800 to $3,000. Your costs will be about double if you get two aids.

Although hearing aids may seem expensive, if they can help you hear better and improve your quality of life, they're worth the investment. Medicare and most private insurance policies don't cover the cost. A few employer- or union-sponsored policies provide limited hearing aid reimbursement. Qualified veterans may be eligible for free hearing aids and services through the Veterans Affairs. Some fraternal and charitable organizations provide financial assistance for hearing aids for people who meet financial eligibility requirements.

Adjusting to a hearing aid

You should notice immediate improvement from wearing a hearing aid, but you'll gain even more benefit after you're accustomed to it. Getting used to a hearing aid takes patience and practice. The brain requires a period of time to adjust to new sounds you haven't heard for a while. Other sounds will seem different when they're amplified by a hearing aid.

To get the maximum benefit from your hearing aid, it's important to understand how it works, learn to insert it properly and then use it regularly. A positive attitude and following through with return appointments also helps. After you've had your hearing aid for a week or two, you may wish to have it adjusted for more or less loudness or for better fit and control. The audiologist or hearing aid dealer will work with you to achieve the best possible fit and hearing.

Your audiologist or hearing aid dealer will continue to counsel you about how to operate, adjust to and maintain the aid. Practice in his or her presence. If you use two aids, insert and remove them to help distinguish between which device is for your right ear and which is for your left ear. Practice adjusting the controls, cleaning the aid and changing the batteries. The dispenser can also advise you on getting the best hearing from your hearing aid.

Readjusting to the world of sounds

When you first use a hearing aid, some sounds may not seem natural. Don't get discouraged. When you've had a hearing loss for a number of years, you've come to think of the way you hear without an aid as normal, even though it isn't. Now when wearing an aid you're exposed to more and louder sounds as well as a different pattern of sounds.

Many first-time users of hearing aids say that other people's voices and their own voices sound strange. The voices are being amplified and heard through a microphone. Hearing aids are often programmed to amplify certain pitches more than others, depending on your hearing loss, so you may be hearing some pitches that you haven't heard for some time. The more you wear your aid, the quicker voices will start to sound normal to you again.

If your hearing has decreased gradually over the years, you've probably become accustomed to a quiet life. Many normal environmental sounds, such as appliance motors, clocks, dripping water, your car's motor and tire noises, footsteps, even your own chewing or breathing, were soft or inaudible without a hearing aid. During the first several months of wearing a hearing aid, you'll notice these sounds again. Because you haven't heard them for a while, your brain is alert to them. They may annoy you. But after several months, your brain will shift them to the background where they belong, and you'll notice the sounds less.

Many hearing professionals recommend that new hearing aid users build up their listening experiences gradually, wearing their aids for only a short time in quiet situations. People often make the mistake of immediately using hearing aids in the most difficult listening conditions, such as a loud restaurant. Starting off in this way can be frustrating and discouraging.

To start the adjustment process, consider using the aid for a few hours a day in your home, where you can control the noise level. Practice conversing with one or two people in a quiet place. Gradually increase the amount of time you use your hearing aid each day. Expose yourself to different listening situations until you're comfortable using your aid all day in any environment. It will take some time, perhaps months, to get used to new sounds and achieve the maximum benefit from your hearing aid.

Discuss problems you encounter with your audiologist or hearing aid dealer. Ask him or her to direct you to a group orientation session for new hearing aid users. This session provides information about hearing loss and hearing aid use. You can also contact an organization such as Self Help for Hard of Hearing People.

Remember that hearing aids are meant to improve communication, not to give you new ears or the hearing of a normal, healthy 20-year-old. You'll inevitably encounter some circumstances in which hearing aids don't give you all of the benefits you'd like. In these situations you can rely on other methods for improving communication, such as those discussed below.

Tips for better communication

Although hearing aids can improve your hearing, they're not a cure-all. In difficult listening situations, consider these strategies to improve understanding:

Talk face to face. Supplement what you hear with what you see. When you're conversing with someone, make sure you can see his or her face and lips. Speak to people on a one-to-one basis or in small groups rather than large groups.

Ask people not to talk to you from a different room. Distance and physical barriers such as walls can reduce the amount of sound that reaches you.

Control background noise. Find locations with the least background noise. Steer clear of noisy restaurants, or go during off-peak times to avoid a crowd. You can also ask for a booth or table in a quiet corner with good lighting. In meeting rooms and lecture halls, sit in the front row. At home turn off the television or stereo during conversation on the telephone or in person.

Ask others to help. People are usually glad to accomodate you when they understand your needs. Let other people know how to help you and what strategies work for you. Start by telling people you have trouble hearing. Ask them to speak clearly, but tell them

Hearing aid batteries

Use only the size and type of battery recommended by your hearing aid dispenser. Most hearing aid batteries are zinc-air. They're activated when an adhesive tab is removed and air gets into the battery. Never remove the tab until you're ready to insert the battery into your hearing aid. Zinc-air batteries have an excellent shelf life, so you can keep several packages on hand. Store them at room temperature, not in a refrigerator.

Battery life depends on the style and circuitry of the hearing aid, the size of battery and how many hours a day the aid is used. Most hearing aid batteries last about one to two weeks. Discuss the battery replacement schedule at your initial fitting.

You can buy batteries from your audiologist or hearing aid dealer, or in drugstores, grocery stores and electronics supply stores. Make sure to keep them out of reach of children and pets, and dispose of them properly.

it's not necessary to shout. Ask them to get your attention by saying your name before they begin speaking to you.

Educate yourself about other hearing tools, such as assistive listening devices. Devices such as a telephone amplifier, FM transmitter, an inductive loop or closed captioning may prove helpful. These devices are discussed in Chapter 9.

Common hearing aid problems

As with any complex piece of equipment, things can go wrong with a hearing aid. Most hearing aid problems are minor and easily corrected. It's important to inform your hearing aid dispenser of these problems. Before calling the dispenser, however, check to make sure the problem isn't something that you can easily fix:

- Is the hearing aid turned on?
- Are all switches or controls in the correct position?
- If you have a remote control for the aid, is it functioning?
- Is the sound outlet plugged with wax or debris?
- Is the microphone opening plugged?
- Is the battery fresh and inserted properly?

Following are some of the most common problems that occur with hearing aids, and ways of solving them.

Feedback. Feedback (whistling) is usually the result of a poor fit, an improperly inserted device or an ear plugged with wax. The more powerful a hearing aid is, the more critical the fit. If your hearing aid whistles, check the following:

- Make sure the aid is inserted properly in your ear.
- Make sure the volume control isn't too high.
- Have your audiologist or doctor check your ear to see if wax has accumulated.

If you wear a hearing aid for some time and feedback becomes a problem, you need to find out if something — such as earwax — is blocking your ear or if your hearing has changed. When in doubt, have your ears examined and hearing tested.

Dead or defective batteries. Weak and faulty batteries are a leading cause of hearing aid failure. Signs of a failing battery are weak output, distortion, increased feedback, and strange or unusual sounds, such as static or fluttering. If any of these signs are evident, try a new battery. Make sure that the battery is inserted correctly with the plus and minus signs facing in the right direction.

Wax blockage. A hearing aid or an earmold in your ear canal seems to stimulate wax production. People who don't wear hearing aids also get wax in their ears, but it gradually loosens, moves to the edge of the ear canal and falls out. With an aid or earmold in place, much of the wax may stay in your ear. Wax can block the loudspeaker and shut it down.

The best way to prevent wax buildup is to visit a doctor or audiologist regularly to have the wax removed. It's a simple procedure. Don't try to remove the wax yourself by using cotton swabs. This will only pack the wax deeper and may damage your eardrum.

Ask your hearing aid dispenser about a means to keep wax from getting inside your hearing aids, such as a wax guard. Every day, inspect the end of the hearing aid where the sound comes out and look for wax blockage. Ask your hearing aid dispenser to show you the best way to clean wax from the aid.

Ear discomfort. Earmolds of a BTE aid should fit snugly but not uncomfortably. In the beginning the earmold may be slightly uncomfortable, but it shouldn't cause soreness, redness or irritation. Ear discomfort can also result from a poorly fitting hearing aid or from an aid that's positioned incorrectly in the ear canal. Difficulties with correct placement are fairly common among many new hearing aid users.

If you experience constant discomfort each time you wear your hearing aids, tell your hearing aid dispenser about the problem. Your earmold or hearing aid may need to be modified or remade.

Moisture. Behind-the-ear hearing aids have the most problems with moisture collecting in the tubing between the earmold and the casing. As warm air from the inside of your ear travels into the cooler tubing, water vapor condenses and collects in the tubing. This usually isn't a problem unless the tubing becomes plugged. Storing the aids in a dehumidifier pack will help.

Taking care of your hearing aid

Proper care is the key to keeping your hearing aid in good working order and ensuring that it'll last as long as possible. Here are some suggestions for maintaining your hearing aid:

Keep your hearing aid clean and dry. Wipe your hearing aid with a tissue or soft cloth every time you take it out of your ear. Gently scrub it with a soft brush every evening when you're done wearing it for the day. A dry, soft-bristle toothbrush works well. Don't wear your aid while bathing, showering or swimming. Keep it away from steamy kitchens or bathrooms where someone has just taken a shower, and don't spray it with hair spray.

Check for wax in the small holes at the tip of the aid. Clean out wax with a small brush, a wire looped around the end of a piece of plastic (a wax loop) or a pick. Consider getting a built-in wax guard on your hearing aid.

Don't expose your hearing aid to intense heat. Don't leave it on the top of a radiator, and don't leave it in the car in the sun.

Store your hearing aid in a safe, dry, dust-free place. You may want to buy a dehumidifying container to store it in at night. Ask your dispenser to recommend a container that would work for you.

Open the battery door when the hearing aid isn't in use. This ensures the hearing aid is off. It also lets air in and moisture out.

Don't drop the hearing aid. Get in the habit of inserting and removing your aid over a soft surface, such as a bed or sofa. Never leave the aid where it could be knocked to the floor.

Have your hearing aid cleaned and serviced regularly. Never repair a hearing aid yourself. This can damage the aid and void the warranty. If the hearing aid breaks or malfunctions, contact your hearing aid dispenser.

Always keep your hearing aid and batteries away from small children and pets. They can choke on an aid or swallow a battery.

Chapter 8

Cochlear implants

Sensorineural hearing loss involves damage to the inner ear and faulty transmission of auditory information to the brain. The damage is often permanent and the hearing loss irreversible. One of the most promising treatments for adults and children with severe to profound sensorineural hearing loss is the cochlear implant. A cochlear implant is an electronic device that provides a sense of sound to people who would get little or no benefit from hearing aids.

A cochlear implant is surgically placed in the inner ear and activated by a device worn outside the ear. It functions something like an artificial inner ear, taking over the job of the cochlea, which translates sounds into electrical signals and sends those signals to the brain for interpretation. A cochlear implant directly stimulates the auditory nerve to send information to the brain.

The first research on cochlear implants began in the late 1950s when scientists began to experiment with ways to compensate for the damaged hair cells in people with sensorineural hearing loss. Since then, cochlear implant technology has evolved to a complex system that's continually improving. Approximately 70,000 people around the world have received implants. In the United States, more than 20,000 people have implants. About half of these are adults and half are children.

Although a cochlear implant doesn't restore normal hearing, it can dramatically improve the ability to hear and to understand speech. Benefits resulting from the surgery vary from one person to another, but most users find that the implant allows them to handle such tasks as talking on the phone. And after someone with a new implant has used the device for a few months, he or she usually finds that the sound of other voices begins to seem natural. For children with hearing loss since birth or a very young age, cochlear implants can help them acquire speech, language and essential developmental and social skills.

Cochlear implants help reduce feelings of isolation and allow people to reap positive social and emotional benefits. Many people with implants feel that their quality of life improves. They're able to enjoy pleasurable sounds such as the rustling of leaves, the cooing of babies and the harmonies of a song. They feel safer because they can hear fire alarms, sirens and traffic noise. They can better perform the tasks of daily living by being able to hear the beep of a microwave and the buzz of a clothes dryer.

Cochlear implants and hearing aids

A cochlear implant is very different from a hearing aid. Hearing aids amplify sounds, making them louder and delivering them to the ear canal. A cochlear implant doesn't make sounds louder. It compensates for damaged or nonworking parts of the inner ear, identifying useful sound information and translating this information into a form that your brain can understand.

Normally, your inner ear converts incoming vibrations from the middle ear into electrical impulses. The delicate hair cells stimulate the auditory nerve to send the electrical impulses to your brain. The brain recognizes the impulses as sound. However, in most people with sensorineural hearing loss, some of the hair cells are damaged and don't function properly. They're unable to stimulate the auditory nerve. Although many nerve fibers may be intact and can still transmit electrical impulses, these fibers are unresponsive because of the hair cell damage.

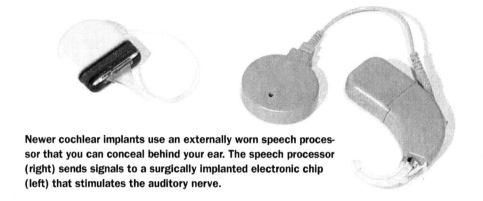

Newer cochlear implants use an externally worn speech processor that you can conceal behind your ear. The speech processor (right) sends signals to a surgically implanted electronic chip (left) that stimulates the auditory nerve.

In people with mild or moderate hearing loss, sounds that are amplified by a hearing aid are converted into electrical impulses by the hair cells that aren't damaged, in the same way that sounds are transmitted in a normal-hearing ear. But if you have profound sensorineural hearing loss, extensive hair cell damage prevents your ears from processing the auditory information, no matter how loud a hearing aid might amplify the sound. Cochlear implants bypass the hair cells and stimulate the surviving nerve fibers in the cochlea. These fibers send electrical signals through the auditory nerve to the brain, allowing you to perceive sound.

How does a cochlear implant work?

Several different cochlear implant systems are available. The Food and Drug Administration (FDA) has approved some and is doing clinical investigations to monitor others. The devices all work by identifying sounds in the environment electronically and sending the impulses to your brain. The implant isn't a single unit but has both internal and external components. The external components are a microphone, speech processor, transmitter and connecting cords. The internal components are a receiver and electrodes. These parts work together as follows:

- The microphone picks up sounds from the environment. It's located in a headset or case worn behind the ear, similar to a behind-the-ear hearing aid.

- A thin connecting cord carries sounds from the microphone to the speech processor, a small, powerful computer that digitally converts the sounds into coded electrical impulses. The coded impulses contain information about the frequency and loudness of the sounds. Speech processors generally come in two styles. One is about the size of a pager and can be worn on a belt or in a pocket. The other is small enough to fit behind the ear. It may be part of the same headset or case that contains the microphone.
- The coded impulses are sent to a transmitter — sometimes called a transmitting coil. A magnet holds the transmitter in place behind the ear, directly over the receiver that's implanted beneath the scalp.
- The transmitter relays the coded impulses as radio waves through the skin to the receiver. The receiver relays the signals to an array of electrodes threaded directly into the cochlea on a bundle of tiny wires.
- The electrodes stimulate nerve fibers in the cochlea that trigger the creation of electrical impulses. This information is sent to the auditory nerve and on to the brain for interpretation.

Although the process seems quite complicated, it all happens very quickly. The length of time between when the microphone picks up a sound and when the brain receives the information is just a few thousandths of a second.

Who can benefit from a cochlear implant?

Cochlear implants aren't an alternative to hearing aids. Rather these electronic devices are designed for individuals who receive little or no benefit from hearing aids. Adults and children who are candidates for a cochlear implant typically have severe to profound sensorineural hearing loss in both ears or have great difficulty understanding speech.

The best age for implantation in children is still being debated, but most children who receive implants are between 1 and 6 years old. The younger a child is at the time of implantation, the less delay there will be in his or her speech and language development, so long as appropriate therapy and education are provided after the implantation.

Among adults, there's no upper age limit for implantation. Several studies have shown that people over age 65 can experience excellent results, gaining significant benefits in both their communication with others and awareness of their environment.

In addition to having some degree of hearing loss, candidates for a cochlear implant must:

- Have realistic expectations — a clear understanding of the benefits and limitations of a cochlear implant
- Be willing and able to make a time commitment for the pre-implant evaluations and postsurgical follow-up services
- Be motivated with the support of family and friends
- Want to be part of the hearing world

The decision to receive an implant should be made only after talking to a cochlear implant audiologist and an experienced cochlear implant surgeon.

Keeping your expectations realistic

Even though thousands of people have received cochlear implants, no one can predict how much benefit any one person will derive from an implant. The varied results depend on a number of factors.

Duration of hearing loss

Adults and children who have experienced a relatively short period of severe to profound hearing loss may adapt to the implant more quickly than may those who have had a profound hearing loss since birth or lost their hearing early in life. For adults, the duration of hearing loss is the foremost predictor of their success with cochlear implants. The shorter the duration, the better the results.

Condition of the auditory nerve fibers

People with a greater number of functioning nerve fibers in the cochlea may benefit more from an implant. Although no test can determine the number or location of surviving fibers, tests such as magnetic resonance imaging (MRI) can indicate whether the cochlea can accommodate implant electrodes.

Motivation and commitment

Much of the success in using a cochlear implant depends on your own motivation and commitment, as well as support from family

---

Cochlear implants and the deaf community

To the surprise of many people in the hearing world, many members of the deaf community strongly object to cochlear implants. People with profound hearing loss often are content in their unique culture, which includes a shared language (American Sign Language), social customs and lifestyle, literature, art, and political, economic and recreational organizations. However, not all people who are deaf participate in this culture.

For many people in the deaf community, deafness isn't regarded as a disorder to be altered. They have an especially negative reaction to implantation in children who are born deaf. Some parents report dealing with unfavorable comments and adverse reactions if they choose an implant for their child.

Some headway has been made in reconciling the two perspectives. Many people recognize the value of being fluent in both worlds. Deaf and hearing-impaired people can continue to use sign language and remain part of the deaf culture while also participating in the larger hearing culture.

Several communication options are available to people with hearing loss, including spoken language and sign language. You may find it helpful to talk with people who have different viewpoints, such as those who use cochlear implants, those who use sign language or both sign and spoken language, and those who oppose implants. Such discussions can help you understand the different perspectives.

By researching your options, you can make an informed decision about the method of communication that's best for you and whether you want to consider a cochlear implant.

and friends. The commitment requires using the implant system full time, maintaining the equipment, keeping follow-up appointments and taking advantage of rehabilitation strategies.

Counseling is an important part of the pre- and post-implantation process. It provides you and your family with realistic expectations about the benefits and limitations of cochlear implants. A cochlear implant is a tool, not a miracle cure. It won't restore normal hearing, but will give you the means to hear.

What defines success with a cochlear implant varies from person to person. Most people who are completely deaf and receive an implant are able to detect medium to loud sounds, including speech sounds, and can learn to recognize familiar sounds. Many users find that cochlear implants help them to communicate better — more than half are able to understand speech without relying on visual cues. In clinical studies of adults who experienced hearing loss after they had learned to speak, 90 percent of the participants reported improved communication without using speech reading. And three-fourths of the participants said they communicated more effectively when at a dinner party, when driving in a car with family members and when ordering at a restaurant. The ability to hear someone calling from another room, to talk on the phone and to enjoy music is within the realm of possibility.

Getting a cochlear implant

An otolaryngologist, commonly known as an ear, nose and throat (ENT) doctor, performs cochlear implant surgery, although not all otolaryngologists perform the procedure. Your doctor can refer you to a cochlear implant center for an evaluation. Cochlear implant centers are located throughout the United States and in many other countries. Before you decide to proceed with implantation, you'll need to undergo a series of tests.

The pre-implantation process
A pre-implantation evaluation will be done by an implant team, which includes an otolaryngologist and an audiologist. The evalua-

tion process can be stopped at any time if you or the implant team feels that it's not appropriate to continue. The evaluation includes the following tests:

Medical evaluation. The ENT doctor will examine the outer, middle and inner ear (otologic examination) to ensure that no active infection or any type of abnormality precludes the use of a cochlear implant. He or she will also do a physical examination to make sure you can safely undergo general anesthesia.

Evaluation with the use of imagery. The doctor reviews your X-rays, computerized tomography (CT) scans or magnetic resonance imaging (MRI) scans to see if the cochlea is suitable for inserting implant electrodes.

Audiologic evaluation. The audiologist performs extensive hearing tests to determine how much you can hear with and without a hearing aid. At the same time, hearing, speech and language tests are conducted to establish a baseline of information for comparison with tests following implantation.

Psychological examination. Some people may need a psychological evaluation to learn if they can cope with the implant and to examine issues that could affect their adjustment to and satisfaction with the implant.

If test results determine that you're a good candidate for implantation, you'll be scheduled for surgery. Before the surgery your implant team will talk with you about the benefits and limitations of implantation, care and use of the equipment, the surgery itself and postsurgical follow-up.

If you or a family member feels anxious about the procedures, feel free to ask questions of the implant team about these concerns.

The surgeon will use these presurgical evaluations to determine which ear to use for the implant. Currently, surgery is done on one ear only — usually the ear with the most severe hearing loss. Research is under way on the benefits of a cochlear implant in both ears, and this may become an option in the future.

Implant surgery
Cochlear implant surgery is performed under general anesthesia and lasts from one to three hours. Your doctor may do the proce-

Cochlear implants and meningitis

The Food and Drug Administration (FDA) is investigating the possibility that cochlear implant recipients may be at a slightly greater risk of bacterial meningitis, an infection of the lining of the brain's surface. Risk of this disease is very small, but because some cases of meningitis have been reported among implant recipients, the FDA is studying whether the design of the implant may be a possible factor. The investigation is being undertaken with the full cooperation of the medical community and cochlear implant manufacturers.

A cause of meningitis in cochlear implant recipients hasn't been established. One theory holds that the implant, because it's a foreign body, might act as a breeding ground for bacterial infection. Some deaf people may have abnormalities of the inner ear that predispose them to meningitis.

If you have or are considering getting a cochlear implant, talk to your doctor about whether you should be vaccinated against organisms that commonly cause bacterial meningitis. In the opinion of the FDA, the American Academy of Otolaryngology — Head and Neck Surgery, and the League for the Hard of Hearing, the cochlear implant remains a safe, effective device that provides many benefits to users. Thousands of people have had cochlear implantation with no adverse side effects.

dure on an outpatient basis, or he or she may have you stay overnight in a hospital.

After anesthesia is administered, the surgeon makes an incision behind the ear and creates a small depression in the skull behind the mastoid bone. The receiver is placed in this depression. A second incision, this one in the mastoid bone, opens up the middle ear. A tiny hole is made in the cochlea, and the electrodes are inserted. A few electronic tests are performed to make sure the device is functioning properly. Then the incision is closed.

When you wake up from anesthesia, you'll find a bulky bandage wrapped around your head to help reduce swelling around the incision. You may experience some pain and nausea. A nurse can offer you medications for either of these effects. On the day of surgery, most people are able to get out of bed for short walks.

The day after surgery, the head bandage is removed. You may be given antibiotics to prevent infection, and most people will take a prescription pain medication for the first three to four days.

Complications of cochlear implant surgery are uncommon. Because the surgery involves your inner ear, your body's balance system may become irritated. This can cause considerable dizziness or vertigo, which will usually improve over the first three to four days, followed by a period of mild unsteadiness for a few weeks. By gently increasing your daily activities, even though you may be slightly dizzy, your balance should gradually return to normal.

Some people report a bitter or metallic taste or other differences in their sense of taste after surgery, which eventually goes away.

Your facial nerve, which controls facial expressions, is located in the area involved in the surgery. Rarely, the nerve may be weakened after surgery, due to temporary swelling. You may notice this if your smile isn't straight or you have trouble closing an eyelid. The condition is treated with cortisone-type medication.

It takes about four to six weeks after surgery for the incision to heal. Most recipients feel well enough to resume their normal activities during this time. However, the cochlear implant will be inactive — it's activated and programmed only after the surgical site heals. Once the skin around the incision heals, the implant is noticeable only as a slight bump.

Activating the implant
After the surgical incision has healed, you'll return to the cochlear implant audiologist for the process of fitting the external components and programming (mapping) the speech processor. During the initial session, a headset or case containing the microphone is placed on your head, and a transmitter is positioned on the side of your head. It's held in place by a magnet that couples with a magnet in the implanted receiver. The speech processor is connected to the microphone and to the audiologist's computer.

One by one, implanted electrodes embedded in the cochlea — each carrying a slightly different frequency or pitch — are turned

A costly procedure

Total costs for getting a cochlear implant — including the pre-implant evaluation, surgery and hospital fees, medical personnel fees, implant hardware and postsurgical fittings and training — can range from $30,000 to $50,000. Unlike hearing aids, cochlear implants are covered by most private insurance plans. Medicare, some state Medicaid programs and the Veterans Affairs provide partial coverage for cochlear implants. In some states, coverage is provided by children's special services, Tricare or state vocational rehabilitation agencies. Many patients have received the support of community or charitable organizations that hold special fundraisers for them, such as the Lions Club, Kiwanis, Sertoma and Jaycees.

The implant center you work with will likely have an insurance or reimbursement specialist who can help you determine the extent of coverage provided by your health plan. He or she can also help you obtain pre-authorization for coverage. It's important that you start the process early and give your insurance company time to review information related to your receiving a cochlear implant.

on. You'll be asked to respond each time you hear a sound and to indicate how loud the sound is. The audiologist uses these measurements to program your speech processor with special computer software. The speech processor is set to the appropriate levels of stimulation for each electrode.

After programming is complete, the speech processor is disconnected from the audiologist's computer. Rechargeable or disposable batteries are inserted into the processor, and you're now able to take the system home.

Your audiologist will work with you to schedule follow-up visits for fine-tuning the speech processor. Repeated adjustments are necessary because it takes time for your auditory nerve to adapt to the signals from the implanted electrodes and for your brain to interpret these signals. As your hearing improves, the speech processor is readjusted.

The time needed to complete the programming of the processor varies among users and among cochlear implant systems. During the first months of implant use, the processor is reprogrammed often. Fewer visits are required after that. Experienced users usually visit their audiologist a few times a year. Schedule a visit to your surgeon and audiologist at least once a year.

Adjusting to a cochlear implant

Everyone who receives a cochlear implant has a different experience with using it. Some adults quickly appreciate sounds they haven't heard for years, and others need a period of adjustment.

Speech heard with a cochlear implant may sound unnatural at first. Over time the sounds will become familiar. The process of adjustment can take anywhere from weeks to years. Adults who haven't had a long period of hearing loss can often rather quickly understand speech without speech reading. Users who have never heard before often need a longer time to adjust to the new sounds.

Learning to listen and make sense of sounds requires a dedicated effort and consistent exposure to sound. Adjusting to a cochlear implant will be easier — and you'll gain more benefit — if you wear the device full time. Start out with easier listening situations, such as conversation with one person in a quiet setting, and work up to more challenging situations, such as groups and places with a lot of background noise. Practice listening to the radio, television and conversation.

Adult users can benefit from various support services. Working with an audiologist, speech-language pathologist or teacher of the hearing-impaired, you can practice identifying sounds, recognizing speech and using speech reading. In addition, training can help you speak more clearly and with good voice quality. The training may include listening-only activities and practice with a telephone. You may be given instructions to continue this training at home.

Rehabilitation training and appropriate education are essential for children who get a cochlear implant. Without such training and education, a child will obtain only partial benefit from the device.

Care and handling

When you get a cochlear implant, members of your implant team will give you detailed instructions about how to take care of the external components. The internal components are designed to last a lifetime. Following are some tips for taking care of your cochlear implant:

- Protect the external components of the system from breakage, moisture and extreme heat.
- On rainy or very humid days, keep a body-worn processor in a plastic bag to protect it from dampness. Watertight pouches are sold at stores that sell scuba-diving equipment. If the speech processor is part of the headset or case, wear a hood when it's raining or snowing.
- Remove the external components before participating in water sports and activities that generate high levels of static electricity, such as using trampolines or plastic slides. Like other electronic devices, cochlear implants can be damaged by static electricity.
- You can wear your implant while participating in most nonwater sports. You don't need to take extraordinary precautions, but it's a good idea to wear protective headgear for activities such as bicycling, in-line skating, football and soccer. Avoid heading a soccer ball.
- Turn off the speech processor before changing batteries, replacing cords or plugging something into it.
- Don't store batteries in the refrigerator. Putting a cold battery in a processor can cause condensation problems.
- Keep the microphone and processor in an anti-humidity kit when not in use.

Children must learn to associate meaning with the new, unfamiliar sounds. They must be taught to understand the sounds and translate them into speech and language.

Speech-language pathologists, educators and family members will need to work together to reinforce the skills that the child is learning. The process takes time, dedication and a lot of hard work.

But throughout childhood, the child's performance will usually continue to improve with the training.

Your audiologist or speech therapist can provide you with other strategies for improving communication and handling difficult listening situations. These strategies are discussed in Chapter 6.

Staying positive

The levels of satisfaction and performance vary among people who receive a cochlear implant. To some extent, personality and psychological factors affect the outcome. For example, whether you're a pessimist or an optimist, whether you have realistic expectations and whether you have a good support network can all influence your progress and satisfaction with the implant.

You can boost your chances of success by keeping a positive attitude. A person who's inflexible and pessimistic may look for — and find — all the wrong things about an implant, regardless of how well it works. In contrast, an optimistic person will focus on the positive improvements he or she is able to make in the long adjustment process. This touches on realistic expectations. If you expect to hear speech clearly in the first few days after your implant is programmed, you'll likely be disappointed.

Having a good support system also is important. Let your family and friends know what they can do to help you succeed with an implant. You can also talk to your audiologist about any problems you're having as you adjust. It's important that at least once a year you return for a checkup at the cochlear implant center or clinic where you had your surgery.

Staying positive doesn't mean that you won't have a range of feelings about the implant. Getting a cochlear implant can trigger many emotions — everyone's reaction is unique. Whatever your experience is, give yourself time to adjust and become used to hearing again. Most people adapt in their own way over time — and find the door to the hearing world open again.

Chapter 9

Other communication aids

Hearing aids and cochlear implants can provide valuable assistance to your hearing if you've experienced hearing loss. But many other options, including assistive listening devices, are available. These devices can help you adapt to different listening environments and allow you to function more effectively with daily tasks.

Much of this relatively new technology can reduce hearing difficulties and solve common problems. It can make life easier and safer — by alerting you when the doorbell rings, by allowing you to listen to television at a reasonable volume, by making telephones easier to use, and by giving you the freedom to participate in many public events and activities.

These communication aids aren't meant to replace hearing aids or cochlear implants. Rather they're intended to augment these devices or enhance your hearing in difficult listening environments, such as noisy restaurants or reverberant lecture halls. Communication aids are also useful for times when you aren't wearing your hearing aid, such as when you're in bed or in the shower. They can alert you to sounds you need to be aware of, such as a smoke alarm, telephone, doorbell or alarm clock.

A variety of communication aids and services are available for use both at home and in public places, including offices, restaurants, hospitals, places of worship, hotels, theaters, airports, trains, buses, libraries and courtrooms. Under the Americans with Disabilities Act (ADA) and other federal legislation, public services and public places are required to make reasonable accommodation for people who are deaf or hard of hearing. This may include different types of communication aids, assistive listening devices, captioning and alerting devices.

This chapter looks at a number of communication devices that connect people who have hearing loss to the larger hearing society. You'll also find information about new developments in science and technology that one day may bring more improvements in hearing and communication.

Difficult listening environments

A sudden, loud noise measuring 140 decibels (db) or more, or a sustained noise exceeding 85 db over an eight-hour period, is hazardous to your hearing. But many situations in daily life at more tolerable noise levels nevertheless can impede your ability to hear and to function effectively. Even if you use a hearing aid, certain situations and environments pose acoustic difficulties. These problem settings include:

- Places with a lot of commotion and background noise, such as restaurants, cafeterias, lobbies, malls, subways and airports. An office can become a noisy place with the sound of foot traffic, manufacturing equipment, printers, copiers, telephones, television and radio.
- Situations where several people may be talking at once, such as parties and social gatherings.
- Large rooms and facilities where the speaker may be far away, such as worship halls, classrooms, theaters and stadiums.
- Locations that are highly reverberant — they easily echo sounds. Places that are likely to be reverberant include those with many hard surfaces, concrete block walls or uncarpeted floors. Examples include classrooms, hallways, basements, open offices, worship halls, arenas and warehouses.

- Situations where a steady, constant background noise is created by a fan, air conditioner, traffic or wind. This type of noise includes the sound of motion on a highway or on rails when you're riding in a car or train.
- Outdoor activities where sound is dispersed, such as sporting events, festivals, parades, picnics and barbecues.
- Telephone conversations, especially when the connection isn't clear. The fact that you can't rely on visual cues can complicate your understanding.

Many of these situations are difficult, if not impossible, to avoid and difficult to plan for. Yet the circumstances often require your active participation as you go about your daily life. Your understanding of what is spoken and your ability to function can benefit greatly from specialized technology developed specifically for these challenging environments.

Assistive listening devices

Assistive listening devices (ALDs) are designed to improve your ability to hear in specific situations in which conventional hearing aids aren't sufficient. These devices can facilitate listening in noisy rooms and in group conversations. They make it easier to use a telephone and hear a distant speaker. In addition, ALDs may be used in one-on-one conversations and for listening to television or radio in the privacy of your home.

ALDs can be used for many social, educational, entertainment and personal activities. Several ALDs are designed for use in large rooms, where people with hearing loss may have trouble understanding the speaker at a podium or on a stage. Frequently, in these settings listeners face problems not only because of distance from the speaker but also because of reverberation and background noise. In classrooms, teachers move back and forth across the room, so the volume of what they're saying may vary. In either of these situations, talking louder may not solve all of your listening problems. Turning up the volume may increase audibility but not necessarily intelligibility.

ALDs work by accentuating or emphasizing the particular sound you want to hear. The goal is to make the desired sound or signal stand out from any background noise. The signal might be a faraway voice, such as a speaker in an auditorium or words coming over a telephone line, or a sound that's closer but gets lost in other noise, such as a companion talking to you in a noisy restaurant. Although ALDs can usually amplify sounds, their primary purpose isn't to make sounds louder. Rather, they place a microphone (pickup) close to the source of the sound you want to hear so that sound becomes clearer and louder compared with other sounds in the environment around you.

Some ALDs are designed for use with hearing aids or cochlear implants, and others are used alone. Many that are used with hearing aids require that the hearing aid have a pickup feature, called the telecoil (t-coil) or telephone switch.

Different ALDs are equipped with a variety of different microphones, headphones, earphones and other features, but they all have two essential parts: a transmitter and a receiver. The transmit-

---

Using your hearing aid's telecoil

Many behind-the-ear and in-the-ear hearing aids are equipped with a telecoil (t-coil). The telecoil is helpful for listening on the telephone. Normally, a hearing aid is sensitive to all sound waves. But when you turn on the telecoil, the aid amplifies only electromagnetic waves from the telephone's receiver. This means that the telephone signal is transmitted directly into the hearing aid without any background noise being amplified.

Most phones are compatible with hearing aids, but when you buy a phone, be sure to ask about hearing aid compatibility. If the salesperson doesn't know, try out the phone before buying it. The telecoil can also be used with FM systems (see page 144) and inductive loop systems (see page 146).

Having a hearing aid with a telecoil broadens your communication options. If your hearing aid has a telecoil and you aren't sure how to use it, consult your audiologist or hearing aid dealer for training.

ter picks up sounds and converts them to signals, then broadcasts the signals. The receiver picks up the signals and carries them to the listener's ears or to hearing aids. Different receivers carried by several individuals can pick up the signal from a single transmitter at the same time.

Telephone devices

Using the telephone can be a challenge for people with hearing impairment. For one thing, listeners can't rely on visual cues to help them with understanding. For another thing, a normal telephone doesn't amplify the sound loud enough for a person with hearing impairment to hear sufficiently. One of the most common and useful ALDs is a telephone amplifier, which may be used with a cell phone or with a wired, cordless or digital phone. The amplifier allows the user to adjust the volume of incoming voices so that even soft voices can be heard more easily.

An amplifier may be installed directly in the telephone or in the handset when the mouthpiece, receiver and buttons are in one unit, or it may be connected as an in-line unit between the telephone and the wall jack. Amplifier handsets are installed in some public telephones, particularly in airports, bus and train stations, museums and hotel lobbies. A telephone access sign identifies the public phones where amplifier handsets are installed.

Portable, snap-on amplifiers are small, battery-operated devices that can be carried in a purse or briefcase and slipped over the receiver of most telephones. Portable amplifiers are helpful for travelers who can't find a public phone with an amplifier handset.

Telephone adapters are portable devices that work with a hearing aid's telecoil. The adapter doesn't amplify sound but instead generates an electromagnetic field that allows the telecoil to pick up the sound directly. An adapter may work with some phones that aren't compatible with portable amplifiers.

Many newer phones don't work with either a telecoil or a portable amplifier, so it's always important to determine beforehand whether a particular phone is compatible.

Other telephone features are available for people with hearing loss. Some telephones have special ringers that produce either an extra loud ring or variable rings to accommodate different types of hearing loss. Visual alerting devices or call indicators can let you know with a flashing light that your phone is ringing. Some phones are equipped for text display of conversations. These devices are discussed in more detail on page 147.

FM systems

You may be familiar with the letters *FM* (frequency modulation) from tuning your radio to a specific frequency in order to hear your favorite FM station. FM systems for the hearing-impaired transmit sounds via radio waves, just like a miniature radio station. They operate on special radio frequencies assigned by the Federal Communications Commission. FM systems are commonly installed in locations where listening may become difficult or large audiences may gather, such as auditoriums, convention centers, places of worship, museums and theaters.

With FM systems, sounds broadcast by a microphone, sound system, radio, television or stereo are directed by a wireless radio

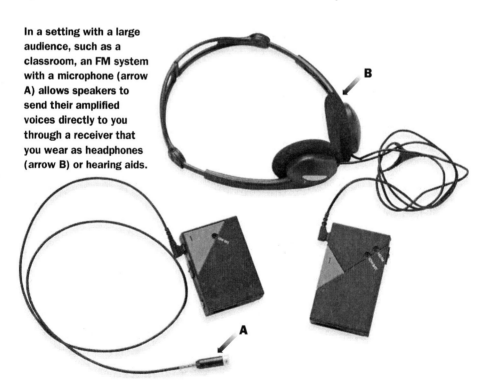

In a setting with a large audience, such as a classroom, an FM system with a microphone (arrow A) allows speakers to send their amplified voices directly to you through a receiver that you wear as headphones (arrow B) or hearing aids.

Buying ALDs and other communication aids

Many assistive listening devices (ALDs) are provided free of charge in public places. If you're planning to buy an ALD or another form of communication aid for personal use, discuss the different options with your audiologist. He or she may have various devices on display. If not, ask for a referral to other locations that would display these devices, including a local audiologic center or speech, language and hearing center, university or college, or community agency for deaf and hard of hearing people.

Communication aids vary in price, so it's wise to comparison shop and work with someone who's knowledgeable about these devices. Check the product's warranty before you buy. Some products come with as much as a five-year warranty.

The staff who dispense ALDs should provide some training, including showing you how to check and recharge batteries.

transmitter to small, portable receivers worn by listeners in the audience who have a hearing impairment.

FM systems can be used with hearing aids that have a telecoil or a direct audio input. To use the telecoil, you wear a small looped cord or necklace of wire that converts the FM signal into electromagnetic waves that are picked up by your telecoil. If you don't have a telecoil, you can link the FM system to a hearing aid using a small adapter called a boot. Several styles of behind-the-ear hearing aids that have a built-in FM receiver are available.

Personal FM systems can be used for one-on-one communication. Composed of a small, portable microphone, receiver and amplifier, they're useful for private conversations in difficult hearing environments such as a busy restaurant or a reverberant auditorium. You can use personal systems while you're walking or in a car, and you can use them to listen to television and radio.

An increasing number of public buildings, government facilities and business offices are being equipped with FM systems to accommodate hearing-impaired visitors. Many schools also are using FM technology for the education of students with hearing impairment.

Infrared systems

Infrared systems for the hearing-impaired transmit sound via light waves to receivers worn by the listeners. Like FM systems, infrared systems are used in locations where hearing is difficult or large groups of people may gather. Infrared technology is also commonly equipped in TV sets for home use.

When this system is used in a large auditorium, an infrared light emitter is plugged into an existing public-address system or sound system. The infrared light waves transmit sound to a portable, lightweight receiver, which may be worn like a headphone by the person with a hearing impairment. Or the receiver can be used with a hearing aid that has a telecoil.

When you use an infrared system with your television, you can set the TV at a volume that's comfortable for others. The infrared transmitter sends the TV signal to your receiver, which you can adjust to as loud a volume as you need. Your adjustments don't raise or lower the volume level used by the others.

With infrared systems, the receiver must be in the transmitter's direct line of broadcast in order to function properly. Sunlight can

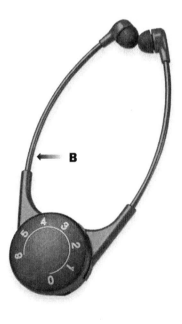

Infrared systems send sounds, for example from a television program, directly to you from a unit that sits on the television (arrow A). A lightweight headset that you wear (arrow B) lets you adjust the device to a volume that you need for hearing while keeping the TV at a volume that's comfortable for others.

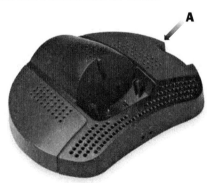

interfere with the transmitter signal, so these systems aren't a good choice for outdoor use. But because the infrared light waves are broadcast along a confined path and not emitted in all directions, infrared systems provide more privacy than FM systems do. Infrared systems are often used in courtrooms and government offices and during live performances in theaters and auditoriums.

Inductive loops

Inductive loop systems, also called audio loop systems, are less commonly used than are FM systems or infrared systems. Inductive loop systems transmit sounds using an electromagnetic field created by a loop of wire installed around the listening area. An amplifier and microphone transmit sound in the form of an electric current that flows through the loop, creating the electromagnetic field. Hearing aids that are equipped with telecoils receive these signals as sounds. Separate receivers can be provided to people who don't have a telecoil feature with their hearing aids.

Inductive loop systems can be permanently installed in the floors of large auditoriums or chambers. Portable loop systems can be set up as needed. Reception with these systems is susceptible to electrical interference.

Telecommunications devices and services

People with very limited hearing or no hearing who can't use a standard telephone can communicate over the phone lines by using text telephones, officially known as telecommunications devices for the deaf (TDDs). They were formerly called teletypewriters and abbreviated as TTYs.

A TDD is a phone with a keyboard. The user types his or her conversation and receives incoming calls as text displayed on a screen or paper printout, sometimes on both. If both callers have TDDs, they each type in their part of a conversation, send it and the text appears on the recipient's text telephone.

A person with a TDD can call someone who lacks a TDD by using the Telecommunications Relay Service (TRS). This free public service allows people who have difficulty hearing or speaking to communicate with people who use standard phones, and vice versa. The Americans with Disabilities Act requires all U.S. telephone companies to provide free relay services to callers throughout the country.

TRS allows real-time conversation by providing a third-party operator, called a communications assistant (CA), who speaks the words typed by a TDD user and types the words spoken by a voice telephone user.

The service is easy to use. Anyone can initiate the call by dialing 711, the number reserved for access to TRS. Communications assistants are available to help you 24 hours a day. The caller provides the CA with the telephone number of the person to be called, and the assistant places the call.

The CA quickly converts each caller's spoken or written words to text or voice. CAs are trained to be unobtrusive and to relay the conversation exactly as it's received. All calls through TRS are confidential. Callers pay only the normal cost of the phone call.

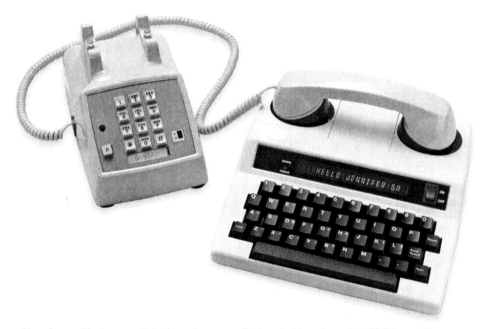

If you're unable to use a telephone because of a hearing impairment, a TDD is an alternative. With a TDD, you can type your conversation and receive a text display of what other people are typing on their TDDs. You can also use a third-party relay service.

When using TRS, a person with a hearing impairment also has the option of speaking directly to the other person and then receiving the response in writing on the TDD, typed by the CA. Another option allows a person with a speech impairment to hear the other party's voice and then relay a TDD response through the CA.

Video relay service (VRS) provides a bridge between people who use sign language and those using spoken English. An interpreter signs back and forth to the sign language user, who communicates via a computer and video equipment. Not all state TRS programs offer this service.

Captioning

Until the early 1970s, some people with hearing loss weren't able to fully enjoy one of America's favorite pastimes — watching television. In 1972, for the first time, a national TV program — Julia Child's cooking show, *The French Chef* — was broadcast with captions that reflected the audio portion of the show. Since that broadcast, captions have opened the world of television to people who are deaf or hard of hearing. Hundreds of hours of entertainment, news, public affairs and sports programming are captioned each week on network, public and cable TV.

Similar to movie subtitles, television captions display dialogue as printed words on the screen. Unlike subtitles, captions also indicate sound effects, music and laughter, and they're carefully positioned to identify speakers. Captions are encoded as data within the television signal, ready for immediate broadcast.

Captions may be displayed as open or closed. Open captions appear on all TV screens and can be viewed without a decoder. Closed captions aren't visible on a standard screen. To display the captions, you need a television with a built-in decoder or a decoder that sits on top of the set. Since 1993, all television sets with screens 13 inches or larger sold in the United States have built-in decoder circuitry. With either form of decoder, you can turn captions on or off with the touch of a button. Because of the widespread availability of closed captioning, open captions are rarely used.

You can tell whether a program has closed captions by the letters *CC* on the screen, often within a television-shaped symbol. Another symbol shows a small TV screen with a tail at the bottom.

Other uses of captioning
Captioning is provided for many movies for sale and rent on DVD and tape as well as for educational and training videos. Captioning is also provided for many live events, such as musical and theater performances, lectures, government proceedings, meetings and conferences. Museums and science centers use captioning in videos and films, demonstrations and planetarium shows.

Some movie theaters offer a captioning system called rear window captioning. An adjustable transparent plastic panel attaches to the viewer's seat and reflects the captions from a panel positioned at the back of the theater.

Alerting devices

A variety of alerting devices are available for someone who is hearing-impaired. Examples of sounds that can be signaled include a telephone ring, a buzz from an alarm clock or kitchen timer, a doorbell, a knock at the door, the cry of a baby, and the sound of a smoke alarm or security alarm.

Alerting devices may use any of three types of signals — an amplified sound, a flashing light or a vibration. For example, an alarm clock can be wired to a vibrating attachment placed under your pillow so that you're gently shaken awake. Or a wake-up alarm with a flashing light can be plugged into your regular alarm clock. Some alerting devices, such as a vibrating personal pager or wristwatch, are designed to get your attention, but they don't necessarily indicate the occurrence of a sound.

Alerting systems can be simple or complex. Some visual alarms use a code to indicate different sounds — for example, a telephone ring might be one light flash, the doorbell three flashes and the smoke alarm regular on-off flashes. Some systems are wired for use in several rooms or from room to room.

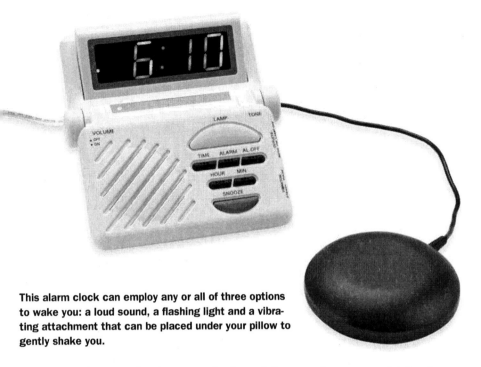

This alarm clock can employ any or all of three options to wake you: a loud sound, a flashing light and a vibrating attachment that can be placed under your pillow to gently shake you.

Some alerting devices are designed for use in your vehicle. A siren alert lets hearing-impaired drivers know when an emergency vehicle is approaching. A blinker buddy tells you that the turn signal is on by flashing a light and sounding an alert that gets louder the longer the signal remains on.

On the horizon

Twenty years ago, hearing aids were just about the only communication aid available for people with hearing loss. Now a wide variety of devices and systems are available, in addition to cochlear implants and improved, more versatile hearing aids. What's more, technology continues to progress. Advances in computer technology, miniaturization and engineering are creating new devices and are making improvements to existing devices. Researchers in a number of fields are searching for new ways to overcome the negative effects of hearing loss and greatly improve communication for millions of people.

Multipurpose communication devices

Imagine wearing a hearing aid that not only improved your hearing but also served as your wireless phone and gave you access to the Internet, voice mail and more. This scenario isn't so far in the future, as advances in computer hardware and electronics create ever smaller processors and as wireless technologies expand.

Researchers are working on fusion products that combine various personal communication devices. These products would look like and function as hearing aids — when needed — but could have many other functions, including a link to telephone, radio and voice mail and a language translator. Various telecommunication devices could be combined with computers and hearing aids by means of technology that uses the body's own electromagnetic field to enable communications between devices.

Speech recognition system

Another area of research and development is speech recognition, also referred to as voice recognition. Speech recognition allows you to control a computer by speaking to it rather than using a keyboard and mouse. You speak commands into a microphone that's connected to the computer. The microphone may be in a headset or mounted on the desktop or a lapel pin.

When a user speaks, his or her commands appear on the computer screen. You can open documents, save changes, delete paragraphs or move the cursor.

The first speech recognition machine was created in 1950. In 1997, continuous-speech-recognition software became commercially available, which means the machine is able to interpret your speaking at a normal conversational rate. These systems are relatively inexpensive and easy to use.

Use of speech recognition software requires training and patience. The speaker has to prepare by entering specialized words into the system's program and training the system to recognize his or her voice patterns. The technology is still not able to handle tricky listening environments. For example, you can't just walk into a noisy party, point a microphone at someone and read his or her speech on a screen.

If you have the proper training, however, speech recognition systems can be very useful. Technology is also being explored as a way to help people who rely primarily on speech reading to communicate. As someone speaks, a computer uses speech recognition and other software to create a sequence of visual cues — hand shapes — that help a speech reader distinguish between different speech elements that look similar when spoken. With video equipment, the cues are superimposed over an image of the speaker's face, allowing the speech reader to follow real-time conversation more easily.

Visual communication systems

Though still in its infancy, visual communication technology has great potential for people with hearing loss, especially those who use sign language as their primary means of communication.

The major system under development involves the use of video and computer equipment to allow people to communicate in sign language over the phone lines or the Internet.

One computer program under development provides real-time translation of spoken or written English into sign language. The hearing party's words are captured by a microphone or inputted as text and displayed on the recipient's computer screen as a signing figure. Another system provides sign language by way of a computer that's fitted with a digital camera and on-call interpreters. A proposed system for communication between two people using sign language converts a speaker's signs to computerized sketches that can be sent to the recipient in a continuous stream, allowing for natural, fluid conversation.

Many options

Many people with hearing loss aren't aware of the numerous options in technology and computer software that can make communication easier. Assistive listening devices and other communication aids can make a huge difference in easing the daily problems caused by hearing loss. It's worthwhile to explore these options. Of course, knowing what might work best for you can be confusing at first, and it's all too easy to be overawed or seduced by the gadgetry. If you're not sure where to start, talk to your hearing health professional, such as your audiologist or ENT doctor.

Chapter 10

Dizziness and problems with balance

The word *dizzy* is used to describe a variety of feelings and sensations — an illusion of motion, lightheadedness, weakness, loss of balance, faintness, wooziness and unsteadiness on your feet. Sometimes, you may feel that you or your surroundings are spinning or whirling. This is commonly called vertigo. Imbalance is the sensation that you must touch or hold on to something in order to maintain your balance.

You may feel dizzy for a number of reasons. Many of them have to do with a disruption somewhere in your complex system of balance. An important part of your system of balance is the vestibular labyrinth, which together with the cochlea, is contained in your inner ear. That explains why some disorders of the inner ear produce both hearing loss and dizziness.

Dizziness is the third most common reason people over age 65 visit their doctor. Aging increases the risk of developing any of the conditions that may cause dizziness. Although it may be temporarily disabling, dizziness rarely signals a serious, life-threatening situation. Doctors can determine the cause of dizziness in about 75 percent of cases, and for most people the signs and symptoms last a short time. Even when no cause is found or the dizziness persists, your doctor can prescribe drugs or other treatments to ease symptoms to a manageable level.

How does your balance system work?

Your system of balance is what allows you to remain upright as you sit, stand or move around. It also keeps your vision clear when your head is moving and keeps you aware of where your head is in relation to the ground.

To maintain your sense of balance, your brain must coordinate sensory information coming from your eyes, musculoskeletal nerves and inner ear. Then the brain sends signals to muscles throughout your skeleton on how to react and maintain your position.

Your vestibular system at work

The vestibular labyrinth is located just above the cochlea in your inner ear. It consists of three loop-shaped, fluid-filled structures called semicircular canals.

At the base of each semicircular canal is a sensory structure called the ampulla. These structures keep your brain informed of the turning motions of your head. This in turn causes your eyes to move in the opposite direction of your head, keeping the image you're looking at focused on the retina.

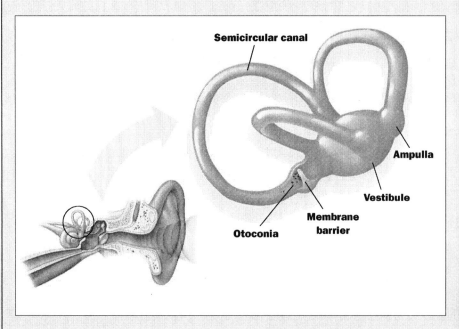

Your eyes. No matter what position you're in — sitting, standing or lying down, moving upright or crouched — visual signals help you determine where your body is in space. When light hits the photosensitive cells at the back of your eyeballs, it triggers chemical reactions that generate electrical impulses. These impulses are communicated to the brain through the optic nerve. Your brain interprets these signals as images, such as the book page in front of you. It also uses these images to calculate, for example, how far your chair seat is above the ground or how fast a car is moving in front of you.

The three semicircular canals are connected to the vestibule. Within the vestibule are two chambers called the utricle and the saccule. The utricle is the upper chamber connecting all three semicircular canals. The saccule is the lower chamber lying closer to the cochlea. These chambers help monitor the position of your head in relation to gravity and to linear motion, such as going up and down in an elevator or moving forward or backward in your car. Each chamber contains a patch of sensory hair cells embedded in a gel-like substance. These patches contain tiny particles called otoconia (o-toe-KOE-nee-uh).

When you bend down to pick something up, the otoconia in the saccule — responsible for the detection of vertical movement — are pulled down by gravity. When you walk forward, the otoconia in the utricle — responsible for detection of horizontal movement — lag behind. In both of these actions, the otoconia pull the gel-like substance with them. This in turn bends the embedded hair cells, causing them to send impulses along their nerve pathways to the brain about your vertical and horizontal movements.

Your brain responds to these impulses, regardless of what you're doing, by coordinating your eye movement with your head movement so that your vision remains clear. Your brain also signals the skeletal muscles to react quickly to help you maintain your balance.

Your system of balance

The brain relays information to and from the eyes, muscles and joints, skin and vestibular labyrinth (within the inner ear).

The eyes record the body's position and surroundings.

The inner ear contains both your primary hearing structure (cochlea) and primary balance structure (vestibular labyrinth).

Muscles and joints report bodily movement to the brain.

When you touch things, sensors in your skin give you information about the environment.

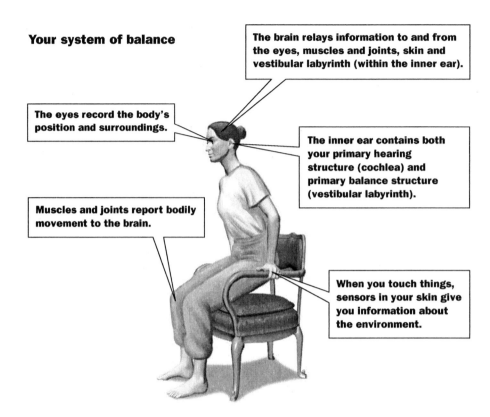

Your nervous system. Millions of nerve cells (neurons) are found in your skin, muscles and joints. When touch, pressure and movement stimulate these cells, they send electrical impulses to your brain about what your body is doing, such as lying on a soft mattress or climbing up a stepladder. Information about the movement of your neck and your ankles is particularly important because it tells your brain which way your head is turned and how steady you are on the ground.

Your vestibular labyrinth. The vestibular labyrinth is the organ of balance contained in your inner ear, alongside the cochlea. Your brain uses the vestibular labyrinth to determine where your head is in relation to gravity and whether your head or body is turning. Although you're not as aware of your vestibular labyrinth as you are of your eyes and musculoskeletal nerves, it's the part of you that your brain relies on most for balance, especially when information from your eyes is missing.

Balance problems can arise from anywhere in this complex system made up of your eyes, musculoskeletal nerves and vestibular labyrinth. In order for you to be able to maintain your balance, at least two of these three sensory systems must be working well. For example, closing your eyes while washing your hair in the shower doesn't mean you'll lose your balance. Signals from your inner ear and musculoskeletal nerves help keep you upright. But if your central nervous system can't process signals from all these locations, if the messages are contradictory or if the sensory systems aren't functioning properly, you may experience a loss of balance.

Causes of dizziness

Everyone has experienced brief episodes of dizziness at one point or another. Momentary dizziness is often caused by rapid changes in your environment. Normally, your sense of balance is maintained subconsciously, based on years of practice and healthy sensory input. For example, a toddler learning to walk is often quite unsteady and frequently loses his or her balance. As you get older, the eye-muscle coordination needed to walk becomes natural, and you don't give it a second thought.

When your brain becomes aware of unusual sensory input — such as your first time on board a boat or when you stand up suddenly after being seated for a long time — you may feel dizzy. The same may happen when you receive conflicting sensory information. For instance, if you're sitting in a theater watching a close-up shot of a speeding train, your eyes are signaling movement while your muscles, nerves and vestibular system indicate you're stationary. This can make you feel dizzy.

Spinning or sudden movements also can cause feelings of dizziness. This happens because the gel-like fluid in your semicircular canals takes a while to catch up with your motion. When you stop moving, the fluid is still going, which makes you dizzy. When the fluid finally comes to rest, the dizziness goes away.

Dizziness caused by environmental changes isn't serious. But sudden, severe attacks or prolonged episodes of dizziness, faintness, lightheadedness or vertigo can be symptoms of an underlying disorder or illness. Sometimes, it's caused by a disturbance of your vestibular system. Other causes may include:

- Low blood pressure. Low blood pressure can make you feel lightheaded or faint when you sit or stand up too quickly.
- Poor circulation. Inadequate blood flow to your brain can make you feel lightheaded. Diminished blood flow to the inner ear may cause you to experience vertigo. Poor circulation may be caused by numerous heart conditions such as blocked arteries, disease of the heart muscle (cardiomyopathy) or irregular heartbeats (arrhythmia).
- Multiple sensory deficits. Lack of input from your eyes, nerves, muscles and joints can make you feel unsteady. Some examples include failing vision, nerve damage in your arms and legs (peripheral neuropathy), osteoarthritis and weakness in your muscles.
- Anxiety disorders. These disorders include panic attacks and fear of leaving your home or being in large, open spaces (agoraphobia). They can make you feel spaced-out or lightheaded.
- Hyperventilation. Abnormally rapid breathing, which often accompanies anxiety disorders, also can make you feel lightheaded or faint.
- Disorders of the central nervous system. These include multiple sclerosis and tumors.

Diagnostic tests

If you see your doctor about a balance problem, he or she may have you undergo several tests to assess the health of your inner ear and balance system. An audiologist usually performs these tests. The results can help determine if one or both ears are being affected, how well your inner ear, eyes, muscles and joints work together to collect sensory information, and whether you may be a candidate for a form of therapy known as vestibular rehabilitation.

You'll likely be asked to not eat, consume alcohol or take any sedatives, tranquilizers, antidepressants or pain relievers for 24

When should you see your doctor about dizziness?
Generally, any unexplained recurrent or severe dizziness warrants a visit to your doctor. Rarely does dizziness indicate a serious illness, but it may happen. See a doctor immediately if you experience vertigo or dizziness with any of the following:
  • New, different or severe headache
  • Blurred vision or double vision
  • Hearing loss
  • Speech impairment
  • Leg or arm weakness
  • Loss of consciousness
  • Falling or difficulty with walking
  • Numbness or tingling
  • Chest pain or rapid or slow heart rate
These signs and symptoms may signal a more serious problem, such as a brain tumor, stroke, Parkinson's disease, multiple sclerosis or heart disease.

hours before testing. You'll also want to wear comfortable clothing, such as pants or a sweat suit, as one of the tests (posturography) requires the use of a harness. The tests aren't dangerous, but they may at times make you feel dizzy, nauseated or anxious. If you have any questions before, during or after a test, be sure to ask your audiologist. An examination may include one or more of the tests described below.

Hearing test
Because the cochlea and vestibular labyrinth are part of the same structure, problems with one often accompany problems with the other. Results of a hearing test can help in the evaluation of your inner ear. For a description of the hearing test, see Chapter 2.

Electronystagmography
Remember how information sent from your vestibular system to your brain controls eye movement while your head is turning? Electronystagmography (ENG) is actually a battery of tests that

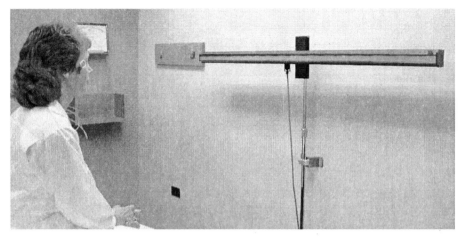

One part of electronystagmography involves watching a light move across a bar. This test evaluates how your eye muscles interact with the balance mechanism in your inner ear.

evaluates the interaction between your inner ear and your eye muscles, known as the vestibulo-ocular reflex. It's considered one of the best ways of checking the balance mechanism of your inner ear.

For the tests, electrodes connected to a computer may be taped to your face. Or you may wear goggles with small infrared cameras mounted to them that constantly track the location of your pupils. In order to determine how well your eye movements respond to signals from your inner ear, you may be asked to:

- Stare continuously at a spot or a light
- Watch a light as it moves across a bar
- Follow rotating spots of light with your eyes
- Lie on a bed in different positions while your eye movements are recorded

Another part of the ENG test is the caloric test, which involves circulating warm water, cool water or air through a soft tube placed in your outer ear canal. Your audiologist will observe your eye movement as the different temperatures stimulate your inner ear.

Dix-Hallpike test

The Dix-Hallpike test is used to determine whether you have a condition known as benign paroxysmal positional vertigo (BPPV). During the test, you'll sit on an examining table while your head is moved to the right or the left at an angle of about 45 degrees. You'll then move quickly from a sitting position to lying down with your head hanging off the back of the table but still at the same angle. You'll be asked to keep your eyes open the whole time so that your audiologist can observe their movement.

If you have BPPV, you'll probably experience vertigo after two to 10 seconds. The sensation may last for 30 seconds to one minute. The procedure is then repeated for the other ear. The ear that's toward the ground when you experience vertigo usually determines which ear is affected. A procedure called canalith repositioning is usually successful in treating BPPV (see page 167).

Rotation tests

Rotation tests also measure your vestibulo-ocular reflex, but they tend to be more sensitive to balance problems that affect both ears. For example, they may be used to monitor your sense of balance while you're taking medications that can cause inner ear problems (ototoxic medications), which typically affect both ears.

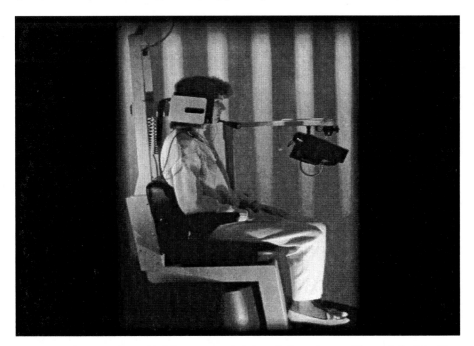

During a rotation test, you'll sit in a rotary chair in a darkened room. The audiologist will monitor your eye movements while your body is rotated in the chair at different speeds and in different directions.

During a rotation test, your audiologist may use electrodes or infrared cameras to monitor your eye movements while your body is rotated in different directions. Often, you will sit in a computer-controlled chair that moves very slowly in a full circle. At faster speeds, it moves back and forth in a very small arc. The testing room is dark most of the time, but a microphone and headset allow you to maintain contact with your audiologist.

Or he or she may have you focus on an object and voluntarily move your head from side to side or up and down for brief periods. In some cases, your audiologist may simply watch your eye movements while he or she moves your head or slowly spins you in a swivel chair.

Posturography
Posturography measures your ability to integrate sensory input from all parts of your balance system, including your eyes, musculoskeletal nerves and vestibular system. This test helps determine which parts of the system you rely on the most and which parts may be giving you problems.

During this test, you'll be asked to stand on a special platform that's sensitive to changes in how you distribute your weight on your feet. This helps to calculate the movement of your center of mass. Then you'll be asked to maintain your balance during conditions in which one or more of your sensory sources are obstructed or altered. For example, you'll be asked to close your eyes or the platform will be put slightly into motion.

This is where comfortable clothes are important because you'll be fitted with a safety harness over your clothes to make sure that you don't fall.

Other tests
A magnetic resonance imaging (MRI) scan can reveal the presence of a tumor or acoustic neuroma. A computerized tomography (CT) scan may be used to check for a temporal bone fracture or other skull abnormalities. Your doctor may also request blood tests to check for infection or cardiovascular tests to check the health of your heart and blood vessels.

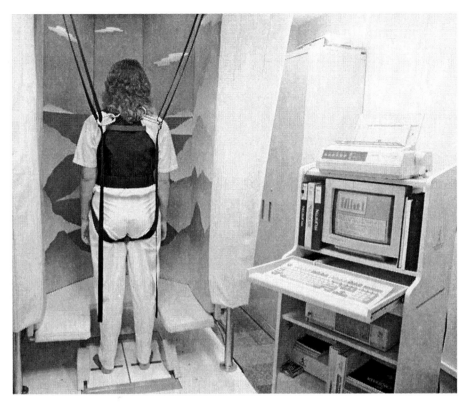

Posturography measures how well you're able to maintain your balance during situations in which conditions have been altered.

Vestibular disorders

Inner ear problems can cause dizziness. Vertigo, in particular — the sensation that you or your surroundings are whirling or spinning — is often associated with vestibular disorders. Problems may arise due to an infection in the inner ear or even to loose otoconia in the vestibular labyrinth.

If you have a vestibular disorder, you may experience nausea or vomiting, changes in heart rate and blood pressure, fear, anxiety and even panic. These effects may make you feel tired or depressed and like you're losing focus. But most of the time, the problem is benign, which means it isn't serious or life-threatening, and your doctor can prescribe ways to manage its signs and symptoms. Some common vestibular disorders are described below.

Benign paroxysmal positional vertigo

Benign paroxysmal (buh-NINE par-ok-SIZ-mul) positional vertigo is commonly known by its abbreviated name BPPV. This condition is a common cause of vertigo, although it's more likely to occur in adults over the age of 50. It's characterized by sudden, short bursts of vertigo — usually lasting less than a minute — that typically occur with changes in head position. You may feel as if you're spinning or floating while lying on one side or the other or with your head tipped back. Your eyes move back and forth involuntarily (nystagmus) when this is happening. You may also experience some nausea with rare occasions of vomiting, and lingering fatigue and queasiness. Vertigo associated with BPPV may come and go unpredictably for weeks or even years.

Although the exact cause is unknown, BPPV is thought to be a natural result of aging, due to gradual degeneration of the vestibular system. Sometimes a blow to the head precedes the condition. Whether the condition is due to aging or trauma, scientists have noticed that the tiny otoconia that normally reside in the utricle of the vestibular labyrinth break loose and, most commonly, accumulate in one of the semicircular canals. Certain movements — such as rolling over in bed, sitting up, looking up or bending forward — may cause the particles to push in on the fluid of the inner ear, bending hair cells and setting off a brief episode of what feels like whirling and spinning.

Anti-vertigo medications

To treat the whirling, spinning sensations of vertigo and curb the nausea that accompanies it, your doctor may recommend or prescribe one of the following medications:
- Meclizine (Antivert, Bonine, others)
- Promethazine (Phenergan)
- Diazepam (Valium)
- Lorazepam (Ativan)

Because these drugs can make you feel drowsy, you may need to avoid operating a vehicle or any sort of heavy equipment after you take them. Also avoid alcohol.

To help relieve benign paroxysmal positional vertigo (BPPV), your doctor may have you use the canalith repositioning procedure, a series of maneuvers that move particles from the semicircular canal back to the utricle. The steps are held for about 30 seconds each. (Movements shown are for the left ear.)

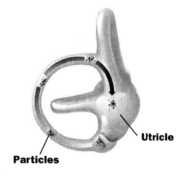

Utricle

Particles

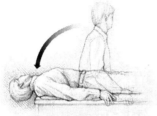

1. Move from a sitting to a reclining position. Head is extended over the end of the table at a 45-degree angle.

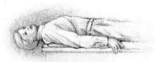

2. Turn your head to the right.

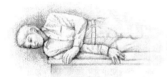

3. Roll over on to your side. Head is slightly angled while looking down at the floor.

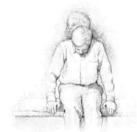

4. Return carefully to a sitting position.
5. Tilt your chin down.

In many cases, a simple procedure may be all it takes to correct BPPV. The canalith repositioning procedure involves simple maneuvers for positioning the head. The goal is to progressively move the misplaced otoconia back to the utricle. It may be necessary to repeat the procedure several times before the feeling of vertigo is eliminated. Afterward, you'll need to keep your head upright for the next 48 hours, even while you sleep. This helps ensure that the particles stay put in the utricle. The success rate when using these maneuvers can be as high as 90 percent, and the signs and symptoms normally don't return. If they do, repeating the procedure usually helps.

Meniere's disease

Meniere's (men-e-AYRZ) disease is an ear disorder that can affect adults at any age. It's characterized by sudden attacks of vertigo, which may last anywhere from 20 minutes to two days and may make you feel nauseated or cause you to vomit. Other signs and symptoms include hearing loss, tinnitus and a feeling that the affected ear is plugged. The vertigo is usually the worst part. Attacks can occur as frequently as every day or as infrequently as once a year. Between attacks, you don't feel any vertigo. Although your ability to hear may fluctuate with the attacks, hearing loss may gradually worsen. Meniere's disease usually affects only one ear, although it may affect both ears in some people.

The exact cause of Meniere's disease is uncertain, but scientists believe it's associated with fluctuation in the volume and content of fluids in the inner ear. Excess fluid can increase pressure on the membranes of your inner ear, distorting and occasionally rupturing them. This can disrupt your sense of balance and hearing.

Treatment of Meniere's disease consists of taking medications to manage the dizziness and nausea and consuming a low-salt diet. Limiting your salt intake can help decrease the level of fluid in your body, including that in your inner ear, and it is hoped, decrease the frequency of attacks. Your doctor may prescribe a diuretic to help accomplish this.

If you experience frequent episodes of vertigo, your doctor may inject a small amount of an antibiotic called gentamicin into your middle ear. Gentamicin is capable of causing inner ear damage, but in controlled quantities it can subdue the activities of the vestibular system and control vertigo while leaving hearing intact. If dizziness is so severe that it inhibits your daily life, inner ear surgery may be an option.

Labyrinthitis

Labyrinthitis is an inflammation of the inner ear, also known as the labyrinth, and may affect both your balance and hearing. The inflammation often follows a bacterial ear infection or a viral upper respiratory illness. It may also occur after a blow to the head, or it may occur by itself, with no other associated illnesses.

Signs and symptoms of labyrinthitis include sudden, intense vertigo that may last for several days, nausea and vomiting, nystagmus, hearing loss and tinnitus. If inner ear inflammation is associated with a bacterial infection, you may experience a total loss of hearing in the affected ear.

To keep the effects of labyrinthitis from getting worse, it's helpful to remain still and avoid sudden changes in position — this is also true of Meniere's disease and vestibular neuronitis. Most of the time, the inflammation goes away on its own after a few weeks, but it's important that you see your doctor. If the underlying problem is bacterial, he or she will likely prescribe antibiotics to get rid of the infectious agent. Steroids are often given if there's no infection. If the condition is diagnosed within 72 hours of onset, your doctor may prescribe antiviral medications. Your doctor may also recommend medications to relieve your dizziness and nausea. In some cases, brief hospitalization is necessary due to dehydration from constant vomiting.

Vestibular neuronitis

Vestibular neuronitis is similar to labyrinthitis in that it causes a sudden onset of vertigo combined with nausea, vomiting and nystagmus. Indeed, the two medical terms are sometimes used interchangeably. Both may be caused by a viral infection, but whereas labyrinthitis is an infection of the inner ear, vestibular neuronitis is an infection of the nerve that leads from the vestibular labyrinth to the brain (vestibular nerve). Because labyrinthitis can also affect the cochlea, it may cause hearing loss. The inflammation caused by vestibular neuronitis does not.

Signs and symptoms may last for days to weeks, being severe at first and then gradually improving. The attack may occur only once, or it may occur several times over a period of a year or more. Often, vestibular neuronitis will develop after a cold or other upper respiratory viral infection. Most people recover completely from the neuronitis, although some may experience a mild imbalance after the infection has resolved. Your doctor may prescribe medications to suppress the vertigo and nausea and steroids such as prednisone to help your body reduce the inflammation. Your doctor may also

Surgery for vestibular disorders

Vertigo and other symptoms of vestibular disorders are most often treated with medications or through rehabilitation therapy, but at times surgery may be an option. This depends on the frequency and severity of your signs and symptoms, the level of your hearing, your overall health and your wishes. Some of the more common surgical procedures for vestibular disorders include:

- Patching a tear in either the oval window or the round window leading from the middle ear to the inner ear (perilymph fistula).
- Placing tissue over a tear at the top of one of the semicircular canals (superior semicircular canal dehiscence).
- Moving a blood vessel that may be pressing up against the vestibular nerve.
- Draining excess fluid (endolymphatic shunt surgery). This operation is performed by draining a sac of fluid (endolymph) that resides near the mastoid bone behind your ear. Sometimes, endolymphatic decompression surgery is performed, which allows more expansion of the endolymphatic sac.
- Cutting the vestibular nerve (vestibular nerve section). The nerve is cut before it joins the auditory nerve to form the eighth cranial nerve. This has the benefit of potentially preserving your hearing while eliminating vertigo. This surgery may be a reasonable option for a younger person with severe symptoms of Meniere's disease and no other significant medical problems.
- Destroying the inner ear (labyrinthectomy). This is a relatively simple operation with fewer risks than in vestibular nerve section. Because it involves destruction of the labyrinth, it's usually reserved for those who have no usable hearing in the affected ear. After the surgery, the brain gradually compensates for the loss of inner ear balance on that side by relying on the unaffected ear for all balance information.

prescribe a form of physical therapy known as vestibular rehabilitation to help in your recovery. This therapy is discussed in more detail starting on page 173.

Reactions to medications

The action of certain medications can damage the organs of hearing and balance in the inner ear. For this reason, these medications are considered ototoxic (*oto* means "ear"). For a list of ototoxic drugs, see Chapter 5. The effects of the medications, which can range from mild to severe, often depend on the dose and the length of time you take them, as well as factors such as kidney and liver function and heredity. With vestibular rehabilitation, someone with a reaction to medications can make remarkable recoveries as the visual system and other systems compensate for the vestibular loss.

If you have an existing balance or hearing problem, or if you experience inner ear problems with certain medications, be sure to let your doctor know. This can help you avoid unnecessary exposure to ototoxic medications. Signs and symptoms of ototoxicity to watch for include:

- Onset of ringing in one or both ears (tinnitus)
- Worsening of existing tinnitus
- A feeling that one or both ears are plugged
- Loss of hearing or worsening of existing hearing loss
- Dizziness or a spinning sensation, sometimes accompanied by nausea
- Loss of balance

Use of alcohol can cause vertigo and nystagmus, which are temporary and go away once the alcohol's effects have subsided. However, the effect of alcohol can last up to 24 hours. Prolonged alcohol abuse can damage parts of your brain and result in permanent imbalance.

Acoustic neuroma

An acoustic neuroma, also known as a vestibular schwannoma, is a slow-growing, benign tumor that develops on the eighth cranial nerve, which is made up of the vestibular and auditory nerves twined together. The tumor develops as a result of overproduction of certain cells, known as Schwann cells, that cover and insulate the nerves. What causes this to develop is uncertain.

Because an acoustic neuroma affects both the vestibular and auditory nerves, hearing loss in one ear, tinnitus, and unsteadiness are common signs and symptoms of the disorder. As the tumor grows, it can affect other nerves that lead to your face, causing facial numbness and facial weakness.

Although an acoustic neuroma generally grows slowly, it's possible for it to grow big enough to push up against the brainstem and interfere with life-sustaining functions. Your doctor may detect the acoustic neuroma with the use of magnetic resonance imaging (MRI). The tumor can be removed surgically or treated with radiation therapy (see Chapter 4).

Perilymph fistula

Perilymph fistula is the medical term for a tear in the membrane covering either the oval window or round window, which are situated between the middle ear and inner ear. It most commonly results from trauma to the head, but may also be caused by rapid changes in atmospheric pressure — such as that experienced while scuba diving or doing airplane maneuvers — and extreme exertion — such as that needed for weightlifting or childbirth.

Signs and symptoms of a perilymph fistula include vertigo, imbalance, nausea and vomiting. A fistula may also lead to tinnitus and hearing loss. Bed rest and avoiding sudden movements often allow the rupture to heal on its own. If this doesn't work, surgery may be performed to repair the opening.

Superior semicircular canal dehiscence

Superior semicircular canal dehiscence (SSCD) is similar to perilymph fistula in that both involve an abnormal opening in the inner ear. With SSCD the abnormal opening is at the top of one of the semicircular canals of the vestibular labyrinth, where there's a lack of bone covering the canal. The primary symptom associated with SSCD is dizziness when straining, for example, when lifting something heavy, or when hearing loud sounds such as dog barks. Treatment may involve surgery.

Vestibular rehabilitation

In many cases, dizziness and vertigo go away on their own. But sometimes they don't. If you experience disruptive signs and symptoms of a vestibular disorder for several weeks or more, your doctor may refer you to a physical therapist for vestibular rehabilitation. This is a therapeutic program that uses specific exercises to decrease your dizziness and help you regain your sense of balance. Vestibular rehabilitation is also frequently recommended after inner ear surgery. It can be a highly effective program, producing 90 percent to 100 percent improvement in some cases.

Compensation

The idea behind vestibular rehabilitation is based on normal, adaptive mechanisms within your brain and central nervous system and musculoskeletal system, which are referred to as compensation. When your vestibular system is damaged, your brain initially receives conflicting messages about your body's movement and position in space, causing dizziness or vertigo. But eventually, your brain goes through an adaptive process in which it resets itself to maximize use of other sources of sensory input in order to make up for the lack of balance information coming from the injured parts. For example, if your inner ear on the left side isn't functioning properly, your balance system will gradually rely more heavily on your right ear to gain the necessary data to maintain your balance. This is compensation.

In order for your brain to be able to compensate, it needs to continue receiving signals from your balance organs, and it needs to be able to adapt. This adaptation often occurs naturally as you continue to move around and carry out your daily activities. When compensation is complete, you rarely feel symptoms of imbalance.

In the beginning, you may try to avoid rapid movement in order to avoid dizziness. But if you continue in a state of inactivity for long periods of time, you may not be providing your brain with the signals it needs to learn new patterns. It's also possible that even with general movement, the brain is simply unable to completely compensate. Anti-vertigo medications play a vital role in relieving acute dizziness, but they are mostly sedative in nature and may, in the long run, delay compensation. Long-term use of anti-vertigo medications is discouraged.

At times the signs and symptoms of a balance disorder become chronic. This can increase your risk of falling and injuring yourself. In older adults, falls are a major cause of disability and death. Thus, vestibular rehabilitation and the prevention of falls may become an important part of your treatment.

What's in a program?

When you enter a vestibular rehabilitation program, the first thing that generally takes place is a thorough assessment of your balance problems. This is done so that your physical therapist can design an exercise program customized especially for you and your needs. A balance assessment typically includes:

- Musculoskeletal evaluation to assess your strength, coordination and flexibility skills
- Balance and gait assessments that are compared with those of others in your age group and that test the interaction of all your balance organs
- Questions about the frequency and severity of your symptoms, when and where they occur, and what factors may trigger an increase in signs and symptoms
- Rating your level of dizziness as you move in and out of various positions

After your therapist has gained a better understanding of your situation, he or she may discuss with you your goals for the therapy, such as improving your eye-muscle coordination and increasing your activity levels, and how you can accomplish them.

Generally, your therapist will show you a number of exercises that you can do at home on a regular basis, in between visits to the physical therapy center. For example, you may be requested to do eye exercises in which you focus on a visual target 10 to 20 feet away while going from a sitting position to a standing position and back again with your eyes open. You may then be asked to repeat the procedure with your eyes closed. Other simple exercises that you can do at home are shown on page 175.

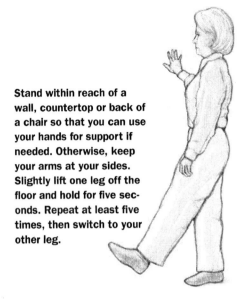

Stand within reach of a wall, countertop or back of a chair so that you can use your hands for support if needed. Otherwise, keep your arms at your sides. Slightly lift one leg off the floor and hold for five seconds. Repeat at least five times, then switch to your other leg.

Place your feet about shoulder-width apart. Raise your hands to your shoulders with your palms facing forward. Extend your right arm and place your left foot forward, pointing down with your toes. Return to starting position and do the same with the opposite arm and foot. Repeat at least five times.

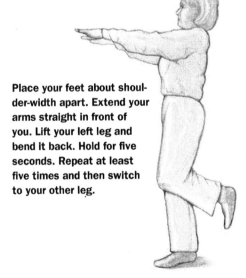

Place your feet about shoulder-width apart. Extend your arms straight in front of you. Lift your left leg and bend it back. Hold for five seconds. Repeat at least five times and then switch to your other leg.

Find a clear hallway and stand at arm's length from the wall so that you can use your hand for support as you walk. Slowly place one foot directly in front of the other and walk heel to toe down the hallway. Repeat at least five times.

These balance-training exercises are intended to hone your balance and coordination skills. Initially, you may want to limit yourself to those exercises that can be done while steadying yourself against a chair or wall. When you become more confident, try the exercises without assistance. Do only those exercises you feel you're able to do safely.

At first, activities like these may make you feel dizzy, and you usually start out doing only a few repetitions at a time. Eventually, however, your brain will become accustomed to these activities — it will find ways to compensate for your vestibular injury — and you'll be able to gradually increase the duration and intensity of the exercises. Your signs and symptoms of dizziness or vertigo will begin to fade away.

You may be given exercises to increase your strength and coordination of muscle responses, to improve your balance control. This might include a daily walking program.

Staying active

Even after you finish the formal therapy program, it's important to keep up your level of physical activity. If your body goes through a period of inactivity, such as during a bout with the flu or after minor surgery, your brain may forget some of its compensation methods, and you may need to retrain your balance system. This can be done readily by regularly performing the exercises that were initially prescribed to you, until the signs and symptoms go away. Generally, they'll recede more quickly the second time around.

Additional resources

Alexander Graham Bell Association for the Deaf and Hard of Hearing
3417 Volta Place N.W.
Washington, D.C. 20007
(202) 337-5220 or (202) 337-5221 (TDD)
www.agbell.org

American Academy of Audiology
11730 Plaza America Drive, Suite 300
Reston, VA 20190
(703) 790-8466 or (800) 222-2336
www.audiology.org/index.php

American Academy of Otolaryngology—Head and Neck Surgery
1 Prince St.
Alexandria, VA 22314
(703) 836-4444
www.entnet.org

American Association of People with Disabilities
1629 K St. N.W., Suite 503
Washington, D.C. 20006
(202) 457-0046 or (800) 840-8844
www.aapd.com

American Auditory Society
352 Sundial Ridge Circle
Dammeron Valley, UT 84783
(435) 574-0062
www.amauditorysoc.org

American Hearing Research Foundation
8 S. Michigan Ave., Suite 814
Chicago, IL 60603-4539
(312) 726-9670
www.american-hearing.org

American Society for Deaf Children
P.O. Box 3355
Gettysburg, PA 17325
(717) 334-7922
www.deafchildren.org

American Speech-Language-Hearing Association
10801 Rockville Pike
Rockville, MD 20852
(800) 638-8255
www.asha.org

American Tinnitus Association
P.O. Box 5
Portland, OR 97207-0005
(503) 248-9985 or (800) 634-8978
www.ata.org

Association of Late-Deafened Adults
1131 Lake St., No. 204
Oak Park, IL 60301
(877) 907-1738 or (708) 358-0135 (TDD)
www.alda.org

Auditory-Verbal International
2121 Eisenhower Ave., Suite 402
Alexandria, VA 22314
(703) 739-1049 or (703) 739-0874 (TDD)
www.auditory-verbal.org

Better Hearing Institute
515 King St., Suite 420
Alexandria, VA 22314
(703) 684-3391
www.betterhearing.org

Canine Companions for Independence
P.O. Box 446
Santa Rosa, CA 95402-0446
(866) 224-3647 or (800) 572-2275
www.caninecompanions.org

Children of Deaf Adults (CODA)
Coda International
P.O. Box 30715
Santa Barbara, CA 93130-0715
www.coda-international.org

Cochlear Implant Association
5335 Wisconsin Ave. N.W., Suite 440
Washington, D.C. 20015-2052
(202) 895-2781
www.cici.org

Dangerous Decibels
Oregon Health & Science University
3181 S.W. Sam Jackson Park Road NRC04
Portland, OR 97201-3098
(503) 494-0670
www.dangerousdecibels.org

International Hearing Society
16880 Middlebelt Road
Livonia, MI 48154
(734) 522-7200
www.ihsinfo.org

National Association of the Deaf
814 Thayer Ave.
Silver Spring, MD 20910-4500
(301) 587-1788 or (301) 587-1789 (TDD)
www.nad.org

National Center for Rehabilitative Auditory Research
3710 S.W. US Veterans Hospital Road
Portland, OR 97207
(503) 220-8262, Ext. 52863
www.ncrar.org/home.htm

National Institute on Deafness and Other Communication Disorders
National Institutes of Health
31 Center Drive, MSC 2320
Bethesda, MD 20892-2320
(800) 241-1044 or (800) 241-1055 (TDD)
www.nidcd.nih.gov

Paws With A Cause
4646 S. Division
Wayland, MI 49348
(616) 877-7297 or (800) 253-7297
www.pawswithacause.org

Self Help for Hard of Hearing People
7910 Woodmont Ave., Suite 1200
Bethesda, MD 20814
(301) 657-2248 or (301) 657-2249 (TDD)
www.hearingloss.org

Vestibular Disorders Association
P.O. Box 4467
Portland, OR 97208-4467
(503) 229-7705 or (800) 837-8428
www.vestibular.org

Glossary

acoustic neuroma. A slow-growing, benign tumor on the auditory and vestibular nerves that develops when cells that cover and insulate the nerves overproduce.

acoustic reflex. A contraction of muscles in the middle ear that helps reduce the effects of a loud sound.

air conduction. How sound waves travel through the ear canal to reach the eardrum.

assistive listening device (ALD). A device designed to highlight a particular sound you're interested in hearing, such as the voice of a distant speaker.

audiogram. A graph produced in an audiometric test that displays the range of sounds you're able to hear.

audiologist. A specialist trained to identify and measure hearing loss, fit hearing aids and help with aural rehabilitation.

auditory brainstem response (ABR). A measurement of the electrical impulses that are sent from the inner ear to the brain when sounds are heard.

aural rehabilitation. Rehabilitation provided by an audiologist or speech-language pathologist that focuses on your adjustment to hearing loss and helps to reduce the difficulties.

behind the ear (BTE). A type of hearing aid with a circuitry casing that rests behind the ear.

benign paroxysmal positional vertigo (BPPV). A condition characterized by sudden, short bursts of vertigo that typically occur with changes in head position.

bone conduction. How sound waves travel through the bones of the skull to reach the inner ear.

caloric test. A test that involves circulating water through the ear canal. The doctor or audiologist observes your eye movement as different water temperatures stimulate your inner ear.

cerumen (earwax). Protective wax in the ear canal.

cochlea. A part of the inner ear that translates incoming sound waves into electrical signals that can be understood by the brain.

cochlear implant. A device that substitutes for damaged hair cells of the inner ear by sending electrical signals to the brain.

completely in the canal (CIC). A small hearing aid in which all parts fit inside the ear canal.

conductive hearing loss. Hearing loss that results from blockage in the ear canal, a ruptured eardrum or restriction of the movement of the tiny bones in the middle ear.

decibel (db). A unit of measure that defines sound intensity based on sound pressure level (db SPL). Decibels also measure how a person's hearing compares with a normal hearing level (db HL).

Dix-Hallpike test. A test to determine whether you have BPPV. The test requires moving quickly from a seated position to lying down with your head at a 45-degree angle.

ear canal. An inch-long pathway leading to the eardrum. The ear canal produces cerumen and contains hairs that prevent bacteria and foreign objects from reaching the eardrum.

earmold. The earpiece of a hearing aid that's made to fit into the ear and direct sound toward the eardrum.

ear, nose and throat (ENT). Physicians in this specialty are known as ENT physicians or otolaryngologists.

electronystagmography (ENG). A battery of tests that evaluate the interaction between your inner ear and your eye muscles.

eustachian tube. A narrow channel that connects the middle ear with the nose and throat.

feedback. A high-pitched whistle or squeal that's made when an amplified sound is picked up by a microphone and re-amplified.

frequency response. The range of frequencies to which a hearing aid can respond, adjusted to your degree of hearing loss.

glomus jugulare tumor. A tumor that may grow in the middle ear and can interfere with vibration of the ossicles.

hair cell. A cell within the cochlea that converts sound waves into electrical impulses that are carried to the brain. Hair cells in the vestibular labyrinth respond to motion.

hearing aid. A device that amplifies sound and directs it into the ear canal.

in the canal (ITC). A type of hearing aid that fits partly in the ear canal but extends to the bowl of the ear.

in the ear (ITE). A type of hearing aid that fills most of the bowl of your ear.

Meniere's disease. A disease characterized by attacks of vertigo and hearing loss that's thought to be caused by a fluid imbalance in the inner ear.

middle ear. An air-filled cavity between the eardrum and inner ear that contains three tiny bones called the ossicles.

mixed hearing loss. A combination of both sensorineural (inner ear) and conductve (middle ear or outer ear) hearing loss.

myringotomy. A procedure in which a doctor will make a small incision in your eardrum to equalize air pressure and remove fluid from your middle ear.

nystagmus. Involuntary back-and-forth movement of the eyes that may accompany vertigo.

ossicle. Any of the three tiny bones (hammer, anvil and stirrup) in the middle ear that vibrate back and forth to transfer sound waves to the inner ear.

otitis media. Middle ear infection, common in children, that occurs when the eustachian tube becomes blocked and the fluid that builds up in the middle ear becomes infected.

otoacoustic emission (OAE). Inaudible but measurable sounds created by the vibrations of hair cells in the cochlea, which bend with the movement of fluid.

otolaryngologist. A doctor trained to diagnose diseases of the ear, sinuses, mouth, throat, larynx and other structures of the head and neck. He or she is also known as an ear, nose and throat (ENT) physician.

otologist. An otolaryngologist who has completed a specialty fellowship focused on ear disorders.

otosclerosis. A condition in which a growth of spongy bone forms around the oval window and stirrup, causing the stirrup to become immobile. Conductive hearing loss results.

ototoxic. A word indicating something that's harmful to your hearing. Ototoxic medications may aggravate an existing hearing problem or cause new hearing problems.

perforation. Damage that results in a hole in the eardrum, often indicated by pain, bleeding or discharge.

posturography. A test that measures how you maintain your balance when one or more of your senses is blocked.

presbycusis. Hearing loss associated with aging that develops when hair cells within your cochlea wear out, causing you to lose sensitivity to sound.

rotation test. A test that monitors your eye movements in relation to your body rotation.

saccule. A chamber in the vestibular labyrinth that helps monitor the position of your head in relation to the ground. The saccule is responsible for detection of vertical movement.

semicircular canal. Any of the three tubes that form the vestibular labyrinth in the inner ear. The canals are filled with fluid and contain hair cells sensitive to fluid movement, which assist with your sense of balance.

sensorineural hearing loss. Hearing loss that results from damage to the inner ear, auditory nerve or brain.

speech reception threshold. The faintest level at which you can understand speech at least half the time.

stapedotomy. A surgery to treat otosclerosis, in which the immobile stirrup is removed and replaced by a prosthesis.

sudden sensorineural hearing loss. Hearing loss in the inner ear that occurs all at once or within only a few days.

telecommunications device for the deaf (TDD). Text telephone that allows people with very limited hearing or no hearing to communicate over the phone.

tinnitus. A sensation of ringing or buzzing in the ears that comes from no apparent source in your surroundings.

tympanic membrane (eardrum). A thin, taut membrane that covers the entrance to the middle ear.

tympanometry. A test that checks the function of the eardrum and middle ear by measuring whether the eardrum moves normally when varying amounts of air pressure are applied to the ear.

utricle. A chamber in the vestibular labyrinth that helps monitor the position of your head in relation to the ground. The utricle is responsible for detection of horizontal movement.

ventilation tube. A small tube inserted into the eardrum that relieves the pressure of a middle ear infection by allowing fluid to drain from the middle ear.

vertigo. An intense feeling that you or your surroundings are spinning or whirling. Vertigo is often due to a problem with your system of balance, which is regulated by the inner ear.

vestibular labyrinth. A structure of the inner ear made up of three fluid-filled, semicircular tubes that assist with balance.

vestibular rehabilitation. A therapeutic program that uses exercises to help you regain your sense of balance.

word recognition testing. A test that determines how well you can hear single-syllable words.

Index

A

Acoustic neuroma, 63–65, 171–172
Acoustic reflex, 12
Acoustic reflex test, 30
Aging and hearing loss, 14, 54-56
Agoraphobia, 160
Airplane ear, 42–43
Alerting devices, 150–151
Alport's syndrome, 69
American Academy of Audiology, 115, 177
American Sign Language 97
American Sign Language Teachers Association, 98
American Speech-Language-Hearing Association, 115, 178
Americans with Disabilities Act (ADA), 88, 98, 140, 148
Amplitude. *See* Intensity
Ampulla, 156
Anatomy of the ear, 4–7
Ankylosing spondylitis, 67
Anvil (incus), 6, 44, 55
Anxiety, 91–92
Anxiety disorders, 160
Assertive communication, 92–93
Assistive listening devices, 141–147

Asymmetrical hearing loss, 33
Atherosclerosis and tinnitus, 74
Audio loop systems, 147
Audiogram, interpreting, 32–34
Audiologists, 19, 114–115
Audiometry, 26–28
Auditory brainstem response test, 30, 31
Auditory cortex, 11, 13
Auditory nerve, 5, 7, 61
Aural rehabilitation, 99–100
Autoimmune inner ear disease (AIED), 66–68

B

Balance problems, 159–176
Balance-training exercises, 175
Barotrauma, 42–43
Basilar membrane, 7, 12
Behcet's syndrome, 68
Behind-the-ear (BTE) hearing aids, 112
Benign paroxysmal positional vertigo (BPPV), 162–163, 166–167
Binaural hearing, 10
Biofeedback and tinnitus, 80
Brain
    and cochlear implants, 126–128

Brain — cont.
  and hearing, 11, 13
  and hearing loss, 15
  and tinnitus, 72

C
Caloric test, 162
Canalith repositioning, 163, 167
Cancer, 48
Captioning, 149–150
Central auditory processing
  disorders, 15
Cerumen (earwax), 5, 14
Cholesteatoma, 47–48
Chronic ear infection, 45–46
Cilia, 7, 12
Circulation problems, 160
Cochlea
  anatomy of, 5, 7
  function of, 11, 12
Cochlear duct, 7
Cochlear implants
  activation process, 134–136
  adjustment period, 136–138
  care of, 137
  controversy, 130
  cost of, 135
  how they work, 126–128
  implant surgery, 132–134
  likelihood of success, 129–131
  and meningitis, 133
  pre-implantation evaluation,
    131–132
  who can benefit, 128–129
Cogan's syndrome, 67
Cognitive therapy and tinnitus,
  79–80

Communication tips, 96–97,
  120–121
Communications assistant, 148
Completely in-the-canal (CIC)
  hearing aids, 111
Computerized tomography
  (CT), 26
Conductive hearing loss
  causes and treatments, 35–52
  defined, 14
  diagnosing, 25, 27–28
Congenital hearing loss, 68–69
Crouzon's disease, 69
Cytomegalovirus, 26, 69

D
Decibels (db), 9, 182
Denial of hearing loss, 87
Depression, 91
Difficult listening environments,
  140–141
Digital hearing aids, 109
Direction of sound, 10
Directional microphones, 114
Disposable hearing aids, 112
Dix-Hallpike test, 162-163
Dizziness, 7, 155, 159–160,
  161, 165
Down syndrome, 69

E
Ear, anatomy of, 4–7
Ear, nose and throat (ENT)
  physicians, 18
Ear canal, 5, 36-40, 47
Ear infection. *See* Middle ear
  infection

Ear protectors, 21, 58–59
Ear specialists, 18–19
Eardrum
  anatomy of, 5
  function of, 12
  perforation of, 28
  retraction of, 28
  rupture of, 40–42
Earmold, 107, 112, 183
Earplugs, 21, 58–59
Earwax blockage, 36–38, 122
Earwax (cerumen), 5, 14
Earwax removers, 38
Electronystagmography (ENG),
  161–162
Endolymphatic shunt surgery,
  170
Eustachian tube, 5, 6, 42

F
Feedback, 110
Fetal alcohol syndrome, 69
Firecrackers and hearing loss, 56
FM listening devices, 114,
  144–145
Foreign object in the ear, 38–39
Frequency of sound
  on an audiogram, 33
  defined, 8

G
Gamma-knife radiation, 64–65
Gene therapy, 70
Glomus jugulare, 48
Glomus tympanicum, 48
Gunshot noise and hearing loss,
  56

H
Hair cell regeneration, 69–70
Hair cells (cilia), 7, 12, 30
Hammer (malleus), 6, 44, 51
Hearing, 10–13
Hearing aids
  adjusting to, 118–120
  battery types, 121
  behind-the-ear (BTE), 112
  care of, 123–124
  common problems with,
    121–123
  completely-in-the-canal
    (CIC), 111
  disposable, 112
  how they work, 106–107
  implantable, 113
  in-the-canal (ITC), 111
  in-the-ear (ITE), 111
  one or two hearing aids, 108
  purchasing, 114–118
  selecting, 107–114
  setting expectations, 104–106
  and tinnitus, 78–79
Hearing dogs, 98–99
Hearing exams
  acoustic reflex test, 30
  adults, 21, 23
  arranging for, 17
  audiometry, 26–28
  auditory brainstem response
    test, 30
  infants and children, 20, 22
  medical history, 23–24
  otoacoustic emissions test,
    30, 31
  physical exam, 24

Hearing exams — cont.
  speech reception test, 28
  tuning fork test, 25
  tympanometry, 28
  word recognition test, 28
Hearing impairment
  and anxiety, 91–92
  aural rehabilitation, 99–100
  coping with, 86–102
  and depression, 91
  and employment, 88–89
  psychological effects, 91–92
  and quality of life, 86–92
  social consequences, 15, 34,
    89–90
Hearing level (HL), 9
Hearing loss
  compensating for, 15
  conductive, 35–52
  due to medications, 65–67
  early signs of, 16
  incidence of, 3–4
  levels of, 29
  noise-induced, 21, 56–59
  prenatal causes of, 26
  sensorineural, 53–69
  sudden deafness, 59
  types of, 13–14
Hearing specialists, 18–19
Hertz (Hz), 8
Hyperacusis, 75
Hyperventilation, 160

I
Implantable hearing aids, 113
In-the-canal (ITC) hearing aids,
  111

In-the-ear (ITE) hearing aids, 111
Identity and self-image, 90
Inductive loop systems, 147
Infrared listening systems,
  146–147
Inner ear
  anatomy of, 7
  common problems of, 53–69
  function of, 12
Insect in the ear, 38–39
Intensity of sound
  defined, 9
  on an audiogram, 33
Internet information, 101
Isolation, social, 90

J
Jaw joint and tinnitus, 76

L
Labyrinthectomy, 170
Labyrinthitis, 63, 168–169
Lead, 67
Lip reading. *See* Speech reading
Loud music and hearing loss, 56
Loudness and hearing damage,
  9, 12, 21, 56–59, 75
Low blood pressure, 160

M
Magnetic resonance imaging
  (MRI), 26
Malignant otitis externa, 40
Manganese, 67
Maskers and tinnitus, 78–79
Medical history, 23-24
Medical specialties, 18–19

Medications
  acyclovir, 59
  Advil (ibuprofen), 39
  Afrin, 43
  alprazolam, 79
  amikacin, 67
  Amikin (amikacin), 67
  Antivert (meclizine), 166
  Aralen (chloroquine), 66
  aspirin, 66
  Ativan (lorazepam), 166
  Auro-Dri, 39
  Aventyl (nortriptyline), 79
  biphosphonates, 51
  Bonine (meclizine), 166
  bumetanide, 66
  Bumex (bumetanide), 66
  carboplatin, 67
  Cardioquin (quinidine), 66
  chloroquine, 66
  cisplatin, 67
  clonazepam, 79
  cyclophosphamide, 68
  Cytoxan (cyclophos-
      phamide), 68
  Dalmane (flurazepam), 79
  Demadex (torsemide), 66
  dexamethasone, 59, 68
  diazepam, 166
  Edecrin (ethacrynic acid), 66
  Enbrel (etanercept), 68
  etanercept, 68
  ethacrynic acid, 66
  flurazepam, 79
  Folex (methotrexate), 68
  furosemide, 66
  Garamycin (gentamicin), 67

gentamicin, 67, 168
ibuprofen, 39
Klonopin (clonazepam), 79
Lasix (furosemide), 66
lorazepam, 166
meclizine, 166
methotrexate, 68
Motrin (ibuprofen), 39
Mycifradin (neomycin), 67
Nebcin (tobramycin), 67
Neo-Synephrine, 43
neomycin, 67
nortriptyline, 79
ototoxicity, 65–66
Pamelor (nortriptyline), 79
Paraplatin (carboplatin), 67
Phenergan (promethazine),
    166
Platinol (cisplatin), 67
prednisone, 59, 68, 169
promethazine, 166
Quinamm (quinine), 66
quinidine, 66
quinine, 66
Rheumatrex (methotrexate),
    68
sodium fluoride, 50
streptomycin, 67
Swim-Ear, 39
tobramycin, 67
torsemide, 66
Valium (diazepam), 166
Vancocin (vancomycin), 67
vancomycin, 67
Xanax (alprazolam), 79
Meniere's disease, 61–63, 76,
    168

Middle ear
anatomy of, 6
common problems of, 43–52
function of, 12
Middle ear infection
(otitis media)
causes and treatment, 44–45
in children, 6, 44
and ruptured eardrum, 40
Mixed hearing loss, 14
Myringotomy, 43

N
N-Butyl alcohol, 67
Nasopharynx, 6
National Board for Certification
in Hearing Instrument
Services, 115
Noise exposure
at home, 60
at work, 21, 23
Noise-induced hearing loss, 21,
56–59, 75
Nystagmus, 166

O
Object in the ear, 38–39
Oil for cleaning ears, 36, 39
Organ of Corti, 7, 53
Ossicles
anatomy of, 6
damage to, 41, 44, 46, 48,
51-52
function of, 12
Ossicular chain disruption,
51–52
Ossiculoplasty, 52

Otitis externa (swimmer's ear),
39–40
Otitis media. *See* Middle ear
infection
Otoacoustic emissions test, 30, 31
Otoconia, 157
Otolaryngologists, 18, 131
Otologists, 18–19
Otosclerosis, 49–51, 76
Otoscope, 24–25
Ototoxicity, 56, 65–67, 171
Outer ear
anatomy of, 5
common problems of, 36–43
Oval window, 6, 49-51

P
Panic attacks, 160
Perforated eardrum, 28
Perilymph fistula, 76, 172
Pinna, 5, 10
Pitch. *See* Frequency
Plasmapheresis, 68
Posturography, 164
Power tools, 56
Presbycusis, 14, 53–56
Pulsatile tinnitus, 74

Q
Quality of life with hearing
impairment, 86–92

R
Radiation treatments, 64–65
Radical mastoidectomy, 47–48
Relationships and social life,
89–90, 92–96

Research directions, 69–70
Resources, 101–102, 177–180
Retraction of the eardrum, 28
Rheumatoid arthritis, 68
Rotation tests, 163–164
Rubella (German measles), 26, 69
Ruptured eardrum, 40–42

S

Saccule, 157
Scala media, 7
Scala tympani, 7
Scala vestibuli, 7
Schwannomas, 76
Scleroderma, 68
Scuba diving and barotrauma, 42–43
Self Help for Hard of Hearing People, 86, 101, 180
Semicircular canals, 7, 156–157
Sensorineural hearing loss
  causes and treatments, 53–69
  defined, 14
Sign language, 97–98
Signs of hearing loss, 16
Sjögren's syndrome, 67
Social isolation, 90
Sodium intake and tinnitus, 76
Sound frequency, 8, 33
Sound intensity, 9, 33
Sound pressure level (SPL), 9
Speech reading, 94–96
Speech reception test, 28
Speech reception threshold, 185
Speech recognition systems, 152–153

Speech spectrum, 33–34
Squamous cell carcinoma, 48
Stapedotomy, 49–51
Stereocilia, 7
Stirrup (stapes), 6, 44, 49, 51
Subjective tinnitus, 74–76
Sudden sensorineural hearing loss (SSNHL), 59
Superior semicircular canal dehiscence, 170, 172
Support groups, 100–101
Surgery
  for cholesteatoma, 47–48
  for chronic ear infection, 46
  cochlear implants, 132–134
  complications, 52
  for ossicular chain disruption, 52
  for otosclerosis, 49–50
  for tumors, 49
  for vestibular disorders, 170
Swimmer's ear, 39–40
Symmetrical hearing loss, 33
Systemic lupus erythematosus (SLE), 68

T

TDD (telecommunications devices for the deaf), 147–149
Tectorial membrane, 7, 12
Telecoils, 114, 142
Telecommunications Relay Service (TRS), 147–149
Telephone amplifiers, 143–144
Television captioning, 149–150
Temporal lobes, 11, 13

Temporary threshold shift, 57
Text telephones, 147–149
Timbre of sound, 10
Tinnitus
from acoustic neuroma, 64
after ear surgery, 52
defined, 71–73
diagnosis, 76–77
and hearing loss, 55, 57, 75
from labyrinthitis, 63
management, 77–82
from medications, 76
medications for, 79
from Meniere's disease, 61
objective vs. subjective, 74
from ruptured eardrum, 41
from tumors, 48
Tinnitus retraining therapy, 81–82
Toluene, 67
Trauma
and hearing loss, 61
and ossicular chain
disruption, 51
and ruptured eardrum, 40–41
Treacher Collins syndrome, 69
Tumors, 48–49
Tuning fork test, 25
Tympanic membrane. *See*
Eardrum
Tympanogram, 30
Tympanomastoidectomy, 46
Tympanometry, 28, 30, 44–45

U
Ulcerative colitis, 67
Usher's syndrome, 69
Utricle, 157

V
Ventilation tube, 45-46
Vertigo, 7, 155, 165-166, 168, 169, 170
Vestibular disorders, 165–172
Vestibular nerve, 7, 61, 171-172
Vestibular nerve section, 170
Vestibular neuronitis, 63, 169, 171
Vestibular rehabilitation, 173–176
Vestibular schwannoma, 63–65
Vestibular labyrinth, 5, 7, 63, 158
Video relay service (VRS), 149
Viral infections, 60–61
Visual communications systems, 153

W
Wegener's granulomatosis, 68
Word recognition test, 28
Workplace issues
hearing impairment, 88–89
noise exposure, 21, 23

MAYO CLINIC ON HEALTH

Alzheimer's Disease

Arthritis

Chronic Pain

Depression

Digestive Health

Healthy Aging

Healthy Weight

Hearing

High Blood Pressure

Managing Diabetes

Osteoporosis

Prostate Health

Vision and Eye Health

Additional Health titles from **Mason Crest Publishers**

COMPACT GUIDES TO FITNESS AND HEALTH

**Alternative Medicine and Your Health
Eating Out: Your Guide to Healthy Dining
Everyday Fitness: Look Good, Feel Good
Getting the Most from Your Medications
Healthy Meals for Hurried Lives
Healthy Traveler
Healthy Weight for Life
Heart Healthy Eating Guide for Women
Live Longer, Live Better
Living Disease-Free
Medical Tests Every Man Needs
Stretching Your Health Care Dollar
Your Guide to Vitamin & Mineral Supplements
Your Healthy Back
8 Ways to Lower Your Risk of a Heart Attack or Stroke
10 Tips for Better Hearing
20 Tasty Recipes for People with Diabetes**